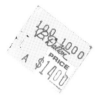

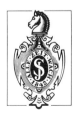

N. Peseschkian

Oriental Stories as Tools in Psychotherapy

The Merchant and the Parrot

With 100 Case Examples for Education and Self-Help

Springer-Verlag
Berlin Heidelberg New York Tokyo

Dr. med. Nossrat Peseschkian
Facharzt für Neurologie und Psychiatrie
Psychotherapie
An den Quellen 1, D-6200 Wiesbaden

Title of the Original German Edition:
N. Peseschkian, Der Kaufmann und der Papagei
© Fischer Taschenbuch Verlag GmbH,
Frankfurt am Main 1979

Title of the Original English Edition:
N. Peseschkian, The Merchant and the Parrot
Vantage Press, Inc., New York 1982

With 15 Figures

ISBN 3-540-15765-4 Springer-Verlag Berlin Heidelberg New York Tokyo
ISBN 0-387-15765-4 Springer-Verlag New York Heidelberg Berlin Tokyo

© Springer-Verlag Berlin Heidelberg 1986
Printed in Germany

Printing and Binding: Offsetdruckerei Julius Beltz, Hemsbach
2119/3140-543210

The Merchant and the Parrot

An Eastern merchant owned a parrot. One day the bird knocked over an oil flask. The merchant became very angry and hit the parrot on the back of the head. From that time on, the parrot, who had previously appeared to be very intelligent, could not talk anymore. He lost the feathers on his head and soon became bald. One day, as he was sitting on the bookshelf in his master's place of business, a baldheaded customer entered the shop. The sight of the man made the parrot very excited. Flapping his wings, he jumped around, squawked, and, to everyone's surprise, finally regained his speech and said, "Did you, too, knock down an oil flask and get hit in the back of the head so that you don't have any hair anymore?"

(After Mowlana)

Contents

List of Stories

For the unity of mankind

Foreword

If you give someone a fish,
you feed him only once.
If you teach him how to fish,
he can feed himself forever.

—Oriental wisdom

When a German or American comes home in the evening, he wants his peace and quiet. That, at least, is the general rule. He sits down in front of the television, drinks his hard-earned beer and reads his newspaper, as if to say, "Leave me in peace. After working so hard, I have a right to it." For him, this is relaxation.

In the East, a man relaxes in a different way. By the time he comes home, his wife has already invited a few guests, relatives, or family and business friends. By chatting with his guests, he feels relaxed, as though freely translating the motto "Guests are a gift from God." Relaxation can thus mean many things. There is no set definition for everything that relaxation comprises. People relax in the way they have learned how, and the way they have learned is what is customary in their family or group, or in the social circle to which they belong.

Just like leisure and relaxation, so customs, habits, and values have many faces. This does not mean that one model is better than the other; rather, it means that various value systems have a lot to say to one another. A set of attitudes developed in one culture can be helpful to persons in another culture. The sustaining motivation for this book is the transcultural view. Over the last thirteen years, I have developed a new concept of psychotherapy and self-education, which has been worked out from a transcultural point of view. I am interested in this transcultural aspect as a result of my own transcultural situation (Germany and Iran). Equally important is my interest in Mideastern stories as resources and communication aids, as instruments in my field of specialization, psychotherapy. An additional factor has been the connection between the wisdom and intuitive thoughts of the Mideast and the new psychotherapeutic methods of the West.

With their playful character and their closeness to fantasy, intuition, and irrationality, stories stand in obvious contrast to the rational and technological models of modern industrial society. The latter's achievement orientation contradicts the essence of stories. Achievement is given priority; the quality of human relationships is relegated to the background; reason and intellect are more highly valued than fantasy and intuition. But we can confront this historically and culturally determined imbalance by supplementing our habitual way of life with different roles and modes of thought, even some that have arisen in a different historical-cultural framework (transcultural starting point). In my work I have tried to explain the universal significance of the transcultural aspect, to systematize the contents of the transcultural problems, and to show its significance for the development of conflicts. With this aspect in mind, I also had another aim, namely to develop a concept for conflict-centered therapy. Different psychotherapeutic methods can be integrated into this short-term therapy according to the indications.

As a Baha'i, I know that such an attempt carries many problems, but I believe that, in the estimates when geographical distances become negligible, such an attempt is useful if not necessary. There is now, in spite of misunderstandings, a hopeful tendency toward unity in diversity. Bahá'u'lláh expressed this with the following verse, the importance of which will again and again shine through this work: "Ye are all leaves of one tree and the fruits of one branch."

Stories that can be used as mediator between therapist and patient are an important help. They give the patient a basis for identification, and at the same time they are a protection for him;

by associating with the story, he talks about himself, his conflicts, and his desires. Especially when there are resistances to be dealt with, the stories have proved their value. Without attacking the patient or his concepts and value directly, we suggest a change of position, which at first has more the character of a game. This change of position finally allows the patient to see his one-sided concepts in relation to others, to reinterpret them and to extend them.

Not Everything at Once

One such story that can help the patient, teachers, parents, and the psychotherapist himself from time to time is the story of the mullah and the riding master.

The mullah, a preacher, entered a hall where he wanted to give a sermon. The hall was empty except for a young groom seated in the front row. The mullah, pondering whether to speak or not, finally said to the groom, "You are the only one here. Do you think I should speak or not?" The groom said to him: "Master, I am but a simple man and do not understand these things. But, if I came into the stables and saw that all the horses had run off and only one remained, then I would feed it nevertheless."

The mullah took this to heart and began to preach. He spoke for over two hours. After that, he felt elated and wanted his audience to confirm how great his sermon had been. He asked, "How did you like my sermon?" The groom answered, "I told you already that I am a simple man and do not understand these things very well. However, if I came into the stables and found all the horses gone except one I would feed it, but I wouldn't give it all the whole fodder I had."

(Oriental Fable)

The fable of the mullah and the groom demonstrates the problems of education and therapy: You either give too little or too much at one time. In both instances, the development of the man is not acknowledged. In stories, myths, parables and concepts, I see a way to allow more room for fantasy and intuition as aids in self-discovery and in the resolution of conflicts.

This "psychotherapeutic" function of stories is the theme of this book. In my previous books, *Psychotherapy of Everyday Life* and *Positive Psychotherapy*, I have already drawn on stories and parables, partly as illustrations for my ideas, but also partly as methods in psychotherapy. The reactions of my readers and my own observations in dealing with my patients led me to wonder what these stories can say to us in the framework of education, self-help, and psychotherapy. But it was not my goal to investigate the contemporary appeal of the stories; instead, I wanted to determine in which conflicts and with which illnesses they could contribute to the solution of problems. It became clear to me that stories have a lot in common with medication. Used at the right time in the right form, a story can become the central point of the therapeutic effort and can lead to changes in attitude and behavior. But, given in the wrong dosage, told in an insincere and moralizing way, its application can be dangerous.

In the eight years that I was involved with stories and compiled the ones contained in this volume, I found again and again that they have something adventurous and unfathomable about them. Thoughts, wishes, and ideas that had been familiar and commonplace to me suddenly appeared in a new light. Other ways of thought that had previously seemed alien now became familiar. It is this change of perspective that I consider to be one of the most essential functions of stories. I hope my readers, too, can participate in the adventure of new points of view and will enjoy the stories.

> *Occasionally we can't avoid science, math and erudite discussions which aid the development of human consciousness.*
> *But occasionally we also need poetry, chess, and stories, so our spirit can find joy and refreshment.*

(After Saadi)

The first part of this book gives an outline of the theory of stories. Proceeding from the ideas of *Positive Psychotherapy*, we will try to determine the functions that stories have in human relationships, particularly in problem-solving and in psycho-therapeutic situations. The second part deals with the practical application of stories. In the first section, we examine the pedagogical meaning of parables in various religions, since religion probably represents the original frame of reference for the stories. The relationship between therapist and patient, as well as its reflection in stories and in the historical descriptions contained in them, is the content of the second segment. The third and fourth segments deal with examples of using stories in therapy. First I discuss problems of sexuality and partnership; then, like a mosaic, an overview of various illnesses, therapeutic questions, and conflicts is given.

Many colleagues who worked with me within the framework of the Psychotherapeutic Discovery group in Wiesbaden (PEW) and the Academy for Continuing Education in the Medical State Association of Hessen have compiled their own observations in using the stories. Many of my patients also contributed to the development of this book by sharing their reactions to the stories. Special mention goes to the teachers' group of the PEW, which discussed the stories and practiced their pedagogical application. At this point I'd like to thank friends and colleagues who gave me suggestions for this book; needless to say, none of them are responsible for the way I have used their suggestions.

I'm indebted to my colleagues, Dieter Schön and Hans Deidenbach, for their creative and critical participation in the preparation and revisions of this book. My secretaries, Mrs. Krieger, Mrs. Kirsch, and Mrs. Hofmann, helped me with their candor, care, and dependability. Through their own transcultural example, my sister, Rezwan Spengler, and my brother, Houchang Peseschkian, gave me many suggestions.

I would like to express my warm thanks to the translator, Mrs. Martha Rohlfing, Chicago.

My wife Manije was a great help in collecting many Mideastern stories, proverbs, and methods of folk psychotherapy as exemplified by my aunt, Mrs. Berdjis, who lives in Iran. My sons, Hamid and Nawid, in the meantime, have also become specialists in the area of Mideastern stories.

Nossrat Peseschkian

Part I

Introduction to the Theory of Stories

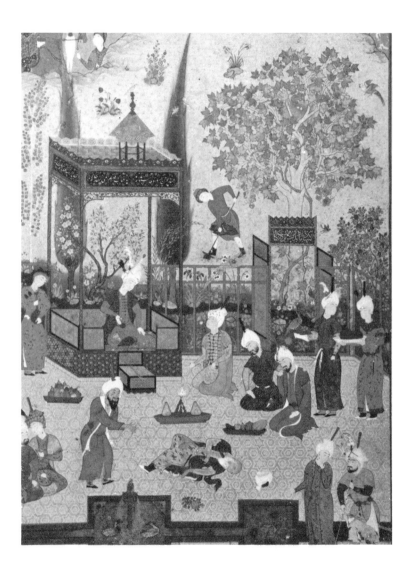

1.

About the Courage to Risk a Test

A king put his court to a test for an important post. Powerful and wise men stood around him in great numbers. "You wise men," said the king, "I have a problem, and I want to see who of you is in a position to solve it." He led the men to a huge door, bigger than anyone had ever seen. The king explained, "Here you see the biggest and heaviest door in my kingdom. Who among you can open it?" Some of the courtiers just shook their heads. Others, who were counted among the wise men, looked at the door more closely, but admitted they couldn't do it. When the wise men had said this, the rest of the court agreed that this problem was too hard to solve. Only one vizier went up to the door. He checked it with his eyes and fingers, tried many ways to move it, and finally pulled on it with a hefty tug. And the door opened. It had just been left ajar, not completely shut, and nothing more had been needed but the willingness to realize it and the courage to act boldly. The king spoke, "You will get the position at the court, for you don't rely just on what you see or hear; you put your own powers into action and risk a test."

In recent years I have compiled a number of Eastern (mostly Persian) myths and fables. I chose these myths because they point to inner conflicts and misunderstandings between people and elucidate the causes and results of these problems. The fact that I turned to Eastern stories is not fundamentally important. In many respects, Eastern and Western myths and wisdoms have common roots; they first became separate as a result of historical-political tensions.

We tend to regard stories, fairy tales, sagas, myths, and parables as the domain of children. There is something old-fashioned about them. The grandmother who tells stories in the West seems to belong to the past as much as does the professional storyteller of the East. This development may have something to do with the fact that stories and myths speak less to reason, clear logic and, hence, to the achievement principle than they do to intuition and fantasy. For a long time, stories were traditionally used in education. They were vehicles by which values, moral views, and behavior models were transmitted and anchored in man's consciousness. Their great entertainment value made them well suited for this. They were the spoonful of sugar that sweetened even the bitterest lesson and made it interesting.

The "moral" of the stories is conveyed in various ways. Sometimes it is immediately apparent; sometimes it is disguised, hidden, or merely hinted at.

2.

Folk Psychotherapy in the Mideast

The Postponement

A man who had been sentenced to death threw himself imploringly at the feet of the hakem, the highest judge. But he found no belief in his words and no witnesses to his innocence. The hakem remained as hard as justice itself. When all the man's pleas proved to no avail, the man asked that his last wish be granted. It's easy, thought the judge, to show a final act of mercy to a man who is facing his death. And, after all, mercy is the best way to ease one's mind about a just act that—as all people know—can go wrong. "What is your wish?" asked the judge. "Lord, my only wish is that I be allowed to utter the two-part prayer {Dorekaat}." The hakem made a gesture of generosity and granted the man's wish. But the man only looked at the judge with fearful eyes. No words came from his lips. The judge lost his patience and asked bruskly, "Why don't you say the prayer?" "Lord," replied the man, "I don't feel safe. Who is to guarantee that the executioner's horrible sword won't chop off my head before I finish my prayer?" "Okay," replied the judge, as he turned to the people who were present. "I swear by Allah and the prophets that nothing will happen to you as long as you haven't finished the prayer." The man fell to his knees, bowed his head toward the East and began his prayer. After the first part, he suddenly jumped up and did not continue praying. "What does that mean?" asked the judge angrily. "Do you want to feel the razor of justice on your neck already?" "Lord, you swore to God that I could utter the two-part prayer before my execution. I have done the first part, and I have just decided to wait to do the second part twenty-five years from now."

In Eastern countries, stories have long been used to teach the lessons of life. This function is tied in with pleasure and pastime. Most of the time, it was storytellers and dervishes who brought stories to the people and thereby helped fill a major need for information, identification, and help in dealing with life's problems. The stories were comprised partly of religious sayings that came from the Koran; others were directly related to human interaction. They took over the function of good advice and harsh measures. People met in coffeehouses, in salons specifically set up for storytelling, or at large family gatherings, mostly on Thursday evening, since Friday is a holiday in the East. Some stories were narrated; others were sung or presented dramatically. Through these approaches, they aroused the feelings of their listeners, for they cried or laughed along spontaneously. As far as I know, this was previously the only public event where men and women—the latter heavily veiled, of course—could participate together.

3.

The Thousand and One Nights

Three Golden Figurines

A king once wanted to test the cleverness and power of discrimination of the neighboring king and the discernment of the king's people. So he sent the king three golden figurines, all with the same appearance and the same weight. The king was supposed to figure out which figure was the most valuable.

Together with his court, the king looked at the figurines, but was unable to see the slightest difference among them. Even the wisest in the land were ready to guarantee that there was no difference. It was depressing for the king to think of the disgrace of having a kingdom where no one was enlightened enough to judge the differing values of the figurines. The whole country participated in this event, and all the people did their best. When they were about to give up hope, a young man sent word from a prison. He would determine the difference if they would just let him inspect the figurines. The king had him brought to the palace and, he transferred the figurines to him. The young man looked them over very carefully. Finally he established the fact that all three figurines had a small hole in the ear. Checking this further, he inserted a thin silver thread. He discovered that, with the first figurine, the thread came out again through the mouth. With the second figurine, the thread came out the other ear. With the third, the thread finally came out through the navel. After thinking about this a while, he turned to the king.

7

"Your highness," he said, "I think the solution to this puzzle lies before us like an open book. We were just supposed to try to read this book. You see, just as every person is different from all others, so each of these figurines is unique in itself. The first figurine reminds us of people who immediately go out and retell what they have just heard. The second figurine is like the person for whom news goes in one ear and out the other. The third figurine, however, is very much like a person who keeps to himself what he hears, and lets it move his heart. Lord! On the basis of this, you should judge the value of the figurines. Which would you want as your confidant? The one who can't keep anything to himself? The one who considers your words no more important than the wind? Or the one who is a trustworthy keeper of your words?"

As an element of folk therapy, stories dealt with inner conflicts long before psychotherapy became a scientific discipline. There are countless examples of how stories were used to deal with life's problems and, in the broadest sense of the word, as psychotherapy. Probably the most well known of these examples is the story collection *1001 Nights,* whose frame story tells how tales were used to help heal a mentally ill ruler. The story can be looked at from two points of view: First of all, there is the successful treatment of the ailing Sultan by the clever Scheherazade. Secondly, the stories are *treatments* for the readers and listeners, as they absorb the contents of the stories, draw lessons from them, and incorporate them into their thoughts. Other stories work in the same way, regardless of whether they come from Eastern, European, or other cultural areas.

Aside from their value as *l'art pour l'art,* such genres as stories, fairy tales, myths, fables, parables, artistic productions, poetry, jokes, and so forth are tools of folk therapy and folk pedagogy, tools with which people helped themselves long before the development of psychotherapy. All of this leads me to the question: Can't these also be used intentionally and consciously in the therapeutic treatment of conflicts and in self-help—all without being dismissed as childish rubbish or nostalgic curiosities, having nothing more than sentimental value? In my medical practice, in seminars, and in lectures, I found again and again that it is primarily parables and

Eastern stories that speak to the listener or patient. For me, they are images in language. They lead to understanding and help develop the ability to empathize.

Many people feel overly burdened when faced with abstract concepts and theories of psychotherapy. Since psychotherapy does not just take place between specialists, but represents a bridge to the patients, the nonspecialists, it is essential that the therapy be comprehensible. Comprehension can be fostered by the mythological story, by the verbal image. It contains the ties to spiritual, human, and social contents and events, and offers possible solutions. Since it is free from the direct world of the patient's experience, and since it does not trigger his resistance to the uncovering of his weaknesses, the mythological example, when used consciously, can help the patient develop a new attitude toward his conflicts. This realization led me to include metaphorical thought as well as mythological stories and fables as aids to understanding in the therapeutic process.

4.

Positive Psychotherapy

The Treasure of Knowledge

A farmer's tractor didn't run anymore. All of the farmer's and friends' attempts to repair it failed. Finally the farmer got to the point where he called for a specialist. The man checked it over, activated the starter, raised the hood, and looked at everything carefully. Finally he took a hammer. With a single blow to a certain part of the motor, he got it back into working condition. The motor hummed as if it had never been out of commission. But, when the farmer saw the expert's bill, he became very angry. "What, you want fifty tuman, when all you did was one blow with the hammer?" "Dear friend," replied the man, "For the blow with the hammer I calculated only one tuman. But I have to demand forty-nine tuman for my knowledge of where the blow had to hit."

Since 1968, I have been working on a new concept of self-help and psychotherapy (differentiation analysis), which I call Positive Psychotherapy. Since the principles and techniques of this method are explained in detail in my book, *Positive Psychotherapy: Theory and Practice of a New Method,* I will give only a short survey here.

Positive Psychotherapy has three aspects:
    a) the positive starting point

10

b) procedures related to the contents
c) the five-phase positive psychotherapy

a) The Positive Starting Point

The term "positive psychotherapy" should point toward
transcultural thinking. In accordance with its original meaning
(Latin *positum*), "positive" means "factual," "given." Illnesses,
disorders, and unsuccessful attempts to solve problems are not the
only things that are factual and given; included among the givens
are the capabilities and potentials that each person has, potentials
that enable him to find new, different, and perhaps even better
solutions. We therefore tried not to cling to the customary
evaluations of conflicts, illnesses, and symptoms. Instead, we tried
to consider other assessments of the problems and to view them in a
new light. It seems especially important to remember that the
patient does not just bring his illness with him; he also brings the
ability to overcome it. It is the therapist's task to help him with
this. In the positive starting point, there is an attempt to work
with the patient to transmit alternative possibilities and solutions,
which, till that time, lay beyond the horizon of consciousness. They
enable us to change our perspective and draw on other models
of thought than those which had kept us more trapped in our
old conflicts in the first place. For example, when our spouse or
friend has been unfaithful, we have many "remedies" at our disposal, each of which produces its own consequences. We can use a
shotgun or knife to reestablish "justice" and "honor." We can
drown our sorrows in alcohol; we can take drugs to find a better
world; we can seek revenge by being unfaithful ourselves. We
can even—usually unconsciously—react physically and try to
solve the problem through somatization, through an "escape
into illness." We can also use discussion to achieve understanding
and insight.
    A similar procedure is applicable for understanding illnesses.
Let's take frigidity as an example. A couple who view it simply as
"sexual coldness" or "the inability to have an orgasm," will

11

experience it differently if other "positive"meanings are taken into consideration.

One such alternative meaning is *frigidity as a way of saying no with one's body*. The effects of this new meaning go beyond simple word play. This interpretation touches on the woman's understanding of herself, the effects of this problem on their relationship, and the way to an eventual treatment. For medicine, for psychotherapy, and also for the potential patient, the positive starting point is thus the catalyst for new ways of thinking.

Stories offer us examples of this process of thinking in new ways. The linearity of logical thought does not lead us out of our problems often enough. In fact, as paradoxical as it may seem, such thought often intensifies the problem. Stories, on the other hand, present solutions that are unexpected and baffling but nonetheless "real" and "positive." Although they seem to contradict logic and custom, they can enable us to take a giant leap out of the cage of our conflicts. The following story illustrates what we mean by a positive procedure.

The situation of a sick person—and not just one who is mentally ill—is in many ways like the situation of a man who stands on one leg for a long time. After a while, his muscles cramp up and the leg that's bearing the weight begins to hurt. But it's not just his leg that hurts; his unusual position causes his entire muscular system to tense up and cramp. The pain becomes unbearable. The man screams for help.

At this point, various helpers come to his aid. While he continues to stand on the one leg, a helper starts to massage it. Someone else begins working on the cramped muscles of his neck. A third helper, noticing that the man is about to lose his balance, offers him his arm as a crutch. Someone in the crowd of onlookers suggests that the man grab hold with both hands, so he can keep standing. A wise old man offers the opinion that the man should realize he's better off than someone who has no legs at all. Another person implores him to imagine he's a feather; the more he concentrates on this image, the more his pains will subside. An enlightened old man who means well adds, "With time, there'll come a solution." Finally a spectator goes up to the wretched man and asks, "Why are you standing on one leg? Straighten out

12

the other one and stand on it. You do have a second leg, you know."

b) Procedures Related to Contents

The Two Halves of Life

A mullah, the proud owner of a boat, invited the village schoolmaster for an excursion on the Caspian Sea. The schoolmaster lolled about under the canopy and asked the mullah, "What kind of weather will we have today?" The mullah checked the direction of the wind, looked up at the sun, wrinkled his brow, and answered, "If you ask me, we's going to have a storm." Horrified by this reply, the schoolmaster made a face and said critically, "Mullah, didn't you ever learn grammar? It's not 'we's,' it's 'we're.'" The mullah responded to this reprimand with nothing but a shrug of his shoulders. "What do I care about grammar?" he asked. The schoolmaster was at his wits' end. "You don't know grammar. That means half your life is down the drain." Just as the mullah had predicted, dark clouds developed on the horizon, a strong wind whipped the waves, and the boat bobbed around like a nutshell. The waves drenched the boat with mountains of water. Then the mullah asked the schoolmaster, "Have you ever learned to swim?" The schoolmaster answered, "No. Why should I learn to swim?" Grinning from ear to ear, the mullah replied, "Well, in that case your whole life is down the drain, because our boat is going to sink any minute now."

In my therapeutic practice I have observed something which I subsequently also found again and again in everyday life (having become attuned to it): In my European, Eastern, and American patients, I have found that symptoms were associated with conflicts that could be traced back to a series of repeated modes of behavior. Generally, I have found that it wasn't big events that led to disorders. More commonly, minor incidents that occurred repeatedly led to sensitive or "weak" spots, which then finally grew into potential conflicts. What was represented as conflict potential and a

13

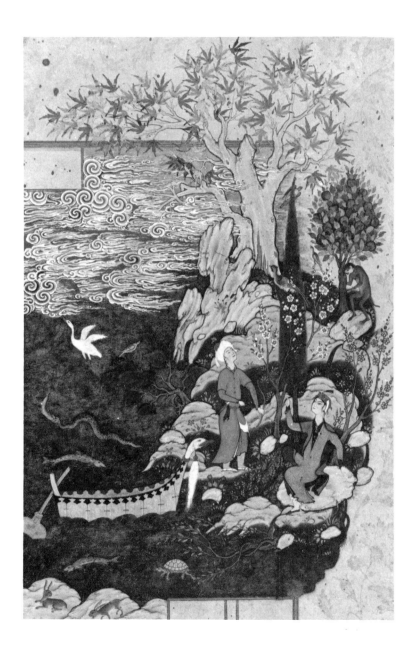

developmental dimension in the educational and therapeutic sectors reappeared as a virtue in the areas of morality, ethics, and religion in a normative sense.

We tried to sort through these areas of conduct and to compile an inventory that would help us describe the substantive components of conflicts and abilities. These areas, which we called "Actual Capabilities," can be divided into two groups. In one group (secondary capabilities), we have the psychosocial norms oriented toward achievement: promptness, order, cleanliness, obedience, politeness, integrity, loyalty, justice, ambition/achievement, frugality, dependability, and precision. In the other group (primary capabilities), we find categories oriented toward feelings: love, patience, time, example, trust, contact, sexuality, hope, faith, unity.

In the course of socialization, the actual capabilities are molded in accordance with the sociocultural value system and are stamped by the unique requirements of individual development. As concepts, they are absorbed into one's self-image and determine how one perceives his environment and deals with its problems. The actual capabilities exert an influence in the following four ways:

1. by means of the senses (relationship to one's body)
2. by means of logic
3. by means of tradition
4. by means of intuition and fantasy (See *Positive Psychotherapy*)

The concepts serve as the helmsmen for our behavior. Let's take for example the concept which is related to the capabilities of "frugality" and "ambition/achievement": If you save something, you have something; if you have something, then you are something. If a person espouses this concept, it will influence his experience and many of his actions: his attitude to his own body, his eating habits, his pleasures, the satisfaction of his needs, his profession, his spouse, his relationships to other people, his fantasies, his creativity, and finally his future. In conjunction with other concepts, this can determine a wide range of individual possibilities, such as "A penny saved is a penny earned," "What counts with me is professional success," or "I need people only for carrying out my own interests," or "Emotions are nonsense; fairy tales are kid stuff."

In this form, the concepts are closely linked to feelings; in the event of a conflict, they can trigger aggression and anxiety. While one person puts a lot of importance on ambition/achievement or on being frugal, another emphasizes orderliness, promptness, relationships, justice, politeness, honesty, and so forth. Each of these norms has its own weight as determined by the situation, the group, and society. These various value orientations confront one another in the course of human contact and in a person's experiences with others. These confrontations can lead to dissonance. The "lively personal disorderliness" of one person, for instance, can be an almost insurmountable problem for someone else who needs a lot of order in his life. In such a case, a person will prefer to change partners than to put up with the other value system and its consequences.

The actual capabilities are very important for positive therapy. In order to test the load capacity of a patient in regard to possible areas of conflict, and to assist him in the differentiation of his situation, we orient ourselves according to a list of actual capabilities, the Differentiation Analysis Inventory—DAI for short.

In this way, we no longer need to speak in general terms about stress, conflict, or illness; instead, we can determine when a conflictual reaction occurs, in which situation, with which partner, and regarding which contents. A woman who regularly suffers severe anxiety attacks when her husband comes home too late at night shows more than just fear of being alone, which would point to the actual capability "contact." Her reaction is also linked to "punctuality." This differentiated procedure enables us to deal more pointedly with the conditions of a conflict.

In stories, the actual capabilities appear in various forms. While pedagogically oriented stories like *Struwwelpeter* mainly convey individual norms such as obedience, politeness and order, other stories challenge these very norms and confront the reader with strange and unusual concepts.

The grouping of the actual capabilities into the secondary capabilities (achievement) and primary capabilities (emotions) is confirmed by a series of findings from brain research. These studies

16

indicate that the two halves of the brain, the two hemispheres, operate according to two separate systems for processing information. The left hemisphere is responsible for logical conclusions, analytical steps, and the verbal components of communication. In other words, the left hemisphere somehow contains the achievement-oriented secondary capabilities and is the representative of understanding and reason. The right hemisphere, which as a rule is not dominant, provides for thinking in totalities, unified comprehension, metaphoric views, and emotional, less-censored associations. The right hemisphere guides the emotionally oriented primary capabilities and is thus the "seat" of intuition and fantasy. Based on this hypothesis, the use of stories and myths in psychotherapy takes on new value: The intended change of perspective comes about because intuition and fantasy are set free. This becomes therapeutically important when reason and rationality alone cannot surmount the problems. One gains entry to fantasy and learns to think in the verbal images of the stories (cf. Watzlawick, et al. 1969).

An almost everyday scene can illustrate the dynamic connection between the actual capabilities and their means of influence. You, the reader, can try to figure out which capabilities determine the course of the following scenario.

A forty-year-old, married businessman is sitting in a train. He's reading the business section of the paper and looks up from time to time to see the landscape flying past his window. At a brief stop, the door to his compartment opens, and a young lady steps in. She's carrying a rather large travel bag, which she then tries to put on the luggage rack. The man lays his paper aside, jumps up, and with a brief "May I?" he gallantly lifts her bag onto the rack. He was already attracted to her the minute she walked in. But, as he sees her sitting there with her legs crossed elegantly, he realizes he's fascinated with her. Suddenly feeling years younger, he bathes in the sunshine of the smile she just gave him for his help. The financial section of the paper no longer interests him. Again and again, he lowers the paper to look at the woman, notices the color of her hair, feels disturbed by the shape and color of her eyes, finds himself looking at her neckline, and tries to concentrate on his

17

newspaper. But he feels caught off guard and under observation. All the while, the most diverse thoughts whirl through his head, thoughts he can't stop.

I like this woman. When I compare my wife with her . . . The phrase "my wife" pulls him back to reality for a minute. *Once upon a time, I was very much in love with her. But since then there's been one problem after another.* Instinctively he recalls that, just the night before, his wife had given him no opportunity to be romantic. Complaining that he showed no other interest in her and was always in such a hurry, she had simply turned her back to him and acted as if she were already asleep. As he thinks of this, he has to gulp, because he sees the woman in front of him. As he catches the scent of her perfume, it seems to him that she's flirting. One thought plants itself in his mind: *I absolutely must get to know this woman. And if I don't botch it up, my wife won't notice a thing. For that matter, how would it be if I traded?* But this isn't an easy idea for him. *Could I actually carry it off? Can I risk it with my kids? What would my relatives say? I'd sure impress my colleagues with an attractive girl friend like that. They'd all like to have one like her.* Suddenly he remembers a scene from his childhood: His mother is crying because her husband has been having an affair. He is stunned by this idea. But he quickly tears himself away from these gloomy thoughts. *I've accomplished a lot in my life and am entitled to get something out of it for a change. All these responsibilities day in, day out. Get up early; flash a smile at my wife (otherwise she gets grouchy); turn in work that's neat and proper and free of error; be friendly to my associates when I'd rather kick them in the ass. Daily aggravation over a thousand petty things.* And, after all that, his wife nagging at night—he can almost hear her voice right now: *"You don't have any time for me. You neglect me. You're not even a real father to the kids."* If that isn't enough to justify his getting to know this fabulous creature sitting across from him, . . . *I deserve it after the dog's life I've had. If only I didn't have these stupid inhibitions.* He holds his paper on his lap, smiles as attractively as he can, clears his throat—and can't produce a sound.

Giving up, he looks out the window. The train slows down, the woman gets up. Before he can lend a hand, she takes her bag from the rack, smiles, and says, "Good-bye." The train pulls into the station. Our businessman watches the woman run toward a young man on the platform. They embrace. The businessman picks up his newspaper and studies the stockmarket as he mutters, "Dumb broad."

c) The Five-Stage Positive Psychotherapy

Give Him Your Hand

A man had sunk into a swamp in northern Persia. Only his head was still sticking out of the morass. At the top of his lungs, he screamed for help. Soon there gathered a crowd of people at the site of the accident. One decided to try to help the poor man. "Give me your hand," he cried over to him. "I will pull you out of the swamp." But the man stuck in the mud just kept crying for help and did nothing to enable the man to help him. "Give me your hand," the man demanded several times. But the answer was always just a wretched cry for help. Then someone else stepped up and said, "Don't you see that he will never give you his hand? You must give him your hand. Then you can save him."

In Positive Psychotherapy, stories are not used randomly, but are chosen within the framework of the five-phase treatment (cf. *Positive Psychotherapy*, 1977). I'd like to illustrate this treatment with an everyday example: When we are mad at someone who has been rude to us, we're inclined to feel upset, to complain openly about him, or to gossip about him and his shortcomings. Suddenly we no longer view him as a person with many capabilities, but only as the rude person, the boor who insulted us. Because these negative experiences overshadow our relationship with this man, we are unable to deal with his other, more positive traits. As a result, we are unable to deal with him; the conflicts remain destructive; communication is limited. This chain of events can lead to psychic and psychosomatic disorders, but, if we use it as a point of departure, we can follow the following phases of a treatment plan:

1. *Observation and Description.* An account is given, preferably in writing, as to the reason for being upset, who caused it, and when.

2. *Inventory.* By using the differentiation analysis inventory (DAI), we determine the areas of conduct where the patient himself and his partner have positive qualities as well as the ones under criticism. In this way, we can counter the tendency toward generalizations.
3. *Situational Encouragement.* To build up a trusting relationship, we strengthen individual traits that we find acceptable and that correspond to the negatively labeled traits.
4. *Verbalization.* To overcome speechlessness or the distortion of speech in the conflict, communication with the partner is developed step by step. There are discussions about positive as well as negative traits and experiences.
5. *Broadening of the Goal.* The neurotic narrowness of perspective is consciously broken down. One learns not to carry the conflict over into other areas. At the same time, one learns to open up new goals that have perhaps never been experienced before. The treatment is thus based on two procedures that run parallel and are intertwined: *psychotherapy,* whereby the relationship between therapist and patient is in the foreground; and *self-help,* whereby the patient takes over therapeutic tasks within the circle of people he is closely involved with.

These are some of the essential steps in differential analytical psychotherapy. Using this methodology, we collected observations in marital conflicts, learning problems, depression, phobias, sexual disorders, and psychosomatic complaints, such as digestive problems, heart and circulatory ailments, rheumatic pains, and asthma. Many cases of psychopathology and schizophrenia were also treated.

The success rate showed that, as a rule, there was a considerable improvement even after a short period (six to ten sessions). In checkup exams a year later, the majority of the cases showed continued success with the therapy. We found especially favorable results in neurotic and psychosomatic disorders. Compared with the other customary forms of therapy, Positive Psychotherapy thus proved to be a favorable alternative.

5.

Transcultural Psychotherapy

A Rooftop Garden and Two Worlds

One summer night, the members of a family slept in the garden on top of their house. To her great displeasure, the mother saw that her son and his wife (whom she barely tolerated anyway) were snuggled up against each other. Unable to bear this sight, she woke them both up and cried, "How can you sleep so close together in this heat? It's unhealthy and dangerous." In another corner of the garden, there slept her daughter and son-in-law, whom she adored. They were sleeping apart from each other, with at least a foot of space between them. The mother woke them up gently by saying, "My darlings, how can you sleep so far apart when it's as chilly as this? Why don't you warm each other up?" The daughter-in-law heard this. She sat up and, with a loud voice, uttered the following words like a prayer: "How mighty is our God. A rooftop garden and such a variable climate."

Transcultural difficulties—in private life, work, and politics—are growing increasingly important today. Given the way society is developing now, the solution of transcultural problems will create one of the major tasks of the future. While people of differing cultural circles used to be separated by great distances and came into contact only in unusual circumstances, technical innovations have dramatically increased the opportunities for contact in

21

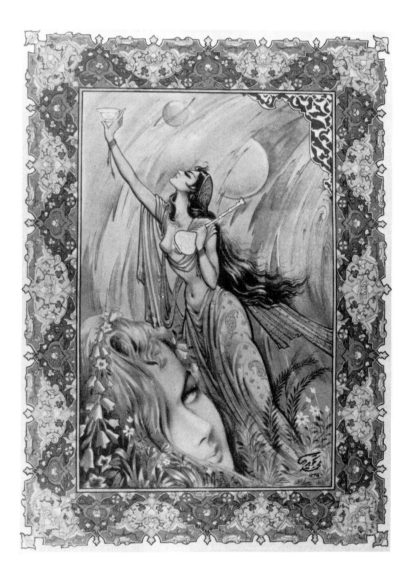

our time. Just by opening the morning paper, we step out of our own living space and make contact with the problems of people from other cultural circles and groups. Generally we interpret these events in ways that we've grown up with. We are ready to criticize, damn, or make fun of them because of their supposed backwardness, naiveté, brutality, or incomprehensible lack of concern.

In the transcultural process, we deal with the concepts, norms, values, behavioral patterns, interests, and viewpoints that are valid in a particular culture.

It is precisely here that we face a danger for transcultural processes (in a double sense of the term): Typification associated with transcultural processes ("the German," "the Persian," "the Oriental," "the Italian," "the Frenchman," and so forth) can lead to stereotyping and prejudice. For this reason it is important always to keep in mind that transcultural descriptions deal with typologies, *i.e.,* with abstractions or statistical relationships that always allow for exceptions and can be refuted by individual cases and historical developments. In this sense, paradoxes are possible, paradoxes we will always encounter, such as "the Prussian Mideastener," who is very serious about punctuality, order, and exactness; or the "Mideast Prussian," whose tolerant and lax attitude toward punctuality makes him well suited for the atmosphere of an Eastern bazaar.

In the same way that there are cultural circles, there are also educational circles within which a person develops his own cultural system, which then collides with other systems. The principle underlying transcultural problem thus becomes the principle for human relationships and the processing of inner conflicts. It thereby becomes an object of psychotherapy.

6.

Stories as Instruments in Psychotherapy

The Half-Truth

The following incident is told about the Prophet Mohammed. The prophet and one of his companions came into a city to teach. Soon an adherent of his teachings came up to him and said, "My lord, there's nothing but stupidity in this city. The inhabitants are so stubborn. No one wants to learn anything. You won't convert any of these hard hearts." The prophet answered kindly, "You're right." Soon after that, another member of the community approached the prophet. Beaming with joy, he said, "Lord, you are in a fortunate city. The people long for the true teaching and open their hearts to your word." Mohammed smiled kindly and again said, "You're right." "Oh, Lord," said Mohammed's companion. "You told the first man he was right, and, with the man who claimed the opposite, you said he was right too. Well, black can't be white." Mohammed replied, "Everyone sees the world as he expects it to be. Why should I refute the two men? The one sees the bad, the other the good. Would you say that one of them sees falsely; aren't the people here and everywhere both good and bad at the same time? Neither of those two men said something wrong, just something incomplete."

Stories can work in many ways. We were interested mainly in those functions that dealt with the origin and evolution of concepts

24

and their educational or therapeutic meaning. In this respect, we stayed with four areas that represented the main centers of conflict: the relationship to one's body; the relationship to achievement/career; the relationship to other people and groups (contact/tradition); and the relationship to intuition, fantasy, and the future.

To prevent a misunderstanding, I must emphasize that we consciously limited ourselves to viewing Eastern stories in their psychosocial function, *i.e.,* in their relevance for the special situation of psychotherapy or for relationships similar to it. In so doing, we work with only one aspect of stories. We leave it to the readers to look at the stories in other ways: to understand them as works of art, as minatures whose meaning is not revealed solely by psychological interpretation.

7.

The Functions of Stories

The Prophet and the Long Spoons

An orthodox believer came to the prophet Elijah. He was motivated by the question of hell and heaven, for naturally he wanted to live his life accordingly. "Where is hell—where is heaven?" As he said these words, he approached the prophet, but Elijah did not answer him. Elijah took the man by the hand and led him through the dark alleys into a palace. They passed through an iron portal and entered a large room crowded with many people, rich and poor, some huddled in rags, some adorned with jewels. In the middle of the room, a big pot of soup, called "asch," stood over an open fire. The simmering casserole spread a wonderful aroma throughout the room. Around the pot, crowds of hollow-cheeked and empty-eyed people jockeyed to get their share of the soup. The man who came along with Elijah was amazed when he saw the spoons the people carried, for the spoons were as big as the people themselves. Each spoon consisted of an iron bowl, white hot from the heat of the soup, and way at the end, a small wooden handle. The hungry people greadily poked around in the pot. Although each wanted his share, no one got it. It was hard to lift the heavy spoon out of the pot, and, since the spoon was very long, even the strongest men could not get it to their mouths. The more impertinent people even burned their arms and faces, or spilled the soup on their neighbors. Scolding one another, they fought and hit each other with the spoons they should have been using to quiet their hunger. The prophet Elijah took his escort by the arm and said, "That is hell!" They left the room and soon were no longer able to hear the infernal cries behind them. After a long journey through dark passages they entered a different room. Here, too, there were many people sitting around. In the middle of the room there was again a pot of hot soup. Each of the persons there had a gigantic spoon in his hand, just like the ones Elijah and the man had seen in hell. But here the people were well nourished. Only a quiet, satisfied humming could be heard along with the sounds of the spoons being dipped into the soup. There were always two people working together. One dipped the spoon in the pot and fed his partner. If the spoon became too heavy for one person, two others helped with their implements so that everyone was able to eat in peace. As soon as one person had had enough to eat, it was another one's turn. The prophet Elijah said to his escort, "That is heaven!"

Stories seem to belong to two different groups:

    a. stories that stabilize the existing norms;

    b. stories that relativize existing norms.

Despite all their contradictions, these two goals are not mutually exclusive. For one thing, the "lessons" of the story depend to a great extent on how the reader reflects on them. And second, the relativization of individual norms, the "change in perspective," does not take place free of values, but in view of other values which the person holds. The reverse is also true. Emphasis on prevailing norms means that other views are called into question or are repudiated. In human interactions as well as in experience and its mental processing, there are certain processes linked to the confrontation with stories. We describe these processes as the "functions" of stories.

The Mirror Function. The abundance of images in stories makes their contents seem closer to the ego and thus helps the reader identify with them more easily. He can project his needs onto the story and can shape its meanings in a way that matches his own psychic structures at that time. These reactions, for their part, can become objects of the therapeutic work. By associating with a story, the patient talks about himself, his conflicts, his wishes. Comprehension and receptivity to the stories are made easier by drawing on the patient's fantasies and memories. Separated from the direct world of experience, stories, if used intentionally, can help lead the patient to a distanced relationship to his conflicts. In this way, he is no longer victim of his illness; he can take a position with regard to his conflicts and to the customary solutions, which are themselves full of conflict. The story becomes a mirror that reflects and can be reflected.

The Model Function. Stories are a model. They reproduce conflict situations and reveal possible solutions, *i.e.,* they point to the results of individual attempts to resolve the conflict. They promote learning by working with the model. But this model is not rigid. It contains a number of possible interpretations and connections to the situation at hand. Stories provide a test situation, where we can try out unusual answers in our thoughts and feelings and then apply them to our conflicts in an experimental way.

The Mediator Function Patients demand a high price for their basic ideas and personal mythologies. Rightly or wrongly, these ideas eventually help them come to terms with existing conflicts. Just as a nonswimmer fears letting go of the inner tube so that he can be hauled into the boat, so the patient is afraid of giving up the ideas that he had used as a lifeline, even though they had maneuvered him into a maelstrom of conflict. This is especially true if a patient is not really sure that the therapist can offer him something of equal or greater value. The patient develops opposition and defense mechanisms that can hinder the therapeutic process on the one hand, but can also provide an entry into the conflict, provided they can be recognized clearly enough.

Resistance can take many forms: silence, tardiness, failure to show up for sessions, doubts about the value of the therapy as expressed through comments about the expense, the demands on one's time, and so on. Such resistance can be dealt with in the therapeutic process. This work, of course, is not necessarily pleasant for the patient. The therapist's *frontal attack* on misconceptions, resistance, and defense mechanisms usually provokes a frontal defense of like intensity.

In the therapy situation, the confrontation between therapist and patient is broken down by the presence of stories as an intermediary between these two fronts. It is a sign of respect for the

or artist who is still permitted to digress from standard norms of achievement and is granted entry to the world of fantasy. Within the therapeutic framework, stories allow the adult to cast off his cloak of acquired behavior and to experiment with fun-loving ideas and attitudes of earlier times. One wants to understand the stories spontaneously, without a lot of afterthought. They open the door to fantasy, to metaphoric thinking, to a fearless and unfettered reaction to fantastic contents, to a sense of awe and wonder. In a way, they transmit *creativity*. They are the intermediary between reality and our desire for pleasure. The stories thus build a bridge to personal wishes and the goals of the near and distant future. Stories make room for utopias, the alternatives to reality.

This descent into earlier developmental periods is guided by the themes in the stories; it allows for some regression—at first only fractional—and enables even the patients with weaker egos to embark on a careful therapeutic process without immediately falling apart. In this connection, I would like to tell about an experience I think was particularly informative.

In a psychiatric clinic, I was leading a mixed psychotherapeutic group where manics participated along with patients suffering from schizophrenic, depressive, and neurotic disorders. Thematically oriented, we started with mythological stories that led to a lively but well-controllable group activity. Even less accessible patients were able to participate to a remarkable degree. This experiment took place in a clinic where analytic psychotherapy in particular was not commonly practiced. Analytical procedures were problematic insofar as it could not be clearly determined in advance that feelings of experience could be controlled within the group.

Stories as Counter-Concepts. By presenting stories, the therapist does not set forth an established theory. He offers the patient a counter-concept that he can accept or reject. In this process, information is consciously placed in a familiar or new situation—in an ambiguous manner, of course. The information can thus intervene one-sidedly into a conflict. Stories are therefore merely an exceptional case of human communication where concepts are also exchanged. An example of this is provided by the following dialog from ancient Persian literature.

31

A tormented father gave his son this advice: "Oh, my son, always abide by the proverb 'Every flower smells different,' and give up all notions of bathing in the manifold deadening blossoms of womanhood." The son gave him cause for thought by saying, "My father, you have not seen the paradisical face of these women. Your eyes have not plunged into the blackness of their hair, and your glance has not rejoiced at the birthmark on their chin, sitting in a corner lost in thought, sinking into sleep while drunk with love, shaken by stormy dreams."

The father responded, "My dear son, you have not seen a table without bread and food. You have not known the harshness of a woman, the crying voices of children, sitting lost in thought in a corner amidst your debts, awaiting the arrival of many unexpected guests."

From this dialog we can assume that father and son have close ties to each other. We sense that, despite their different points of view, there are points of contact between them. Neither can expect a change to occur immediately or, better said, here and now. Their positions are clarified; information is transmitted back and forth and, from all appearances, is understood. But first the information has to be tested to see whether it fits their concepts, or whether it is so compelling that one of the two might alter his original concept. One identifies with the new views temporarily or on an experimental basis and determines what parts are acceptable, what parts can help create a better grasp of reality, and what must be discarded as inapplicable. In other words, both persons in the conversation need time before they can draw results from the new information.

In the psychotherapeutic situation, counter-concepts are offered as prescriptions. The patient is given the task of working with the counter-concept. This can mean that the patient should read a story, think about it, talk about it, or write down his understanding of it. The therapist can expressly prescribe this assignment or—without specifically mentioning it—he can let the challenging quality of the story lead the patient to practice the counter-concept. The form of the counter-concept likewise depends on the circumstances. One can choose from such forms as stories that transcribe the information with a lot of redundancy and poetic imagery; selections where the "moral of the story" briefly summarizes the informative concept; a proverb or saying that conveys the idea; a "formless" counter-concept, which develops directly as an answer to what the patient has to offer.

Change of Perspective. Most of our stories go beyond pure description and contain a reverse experience such as we know from optical illusions. Without expending a lot of effort, the hearer or listener gains a change of perspective, which comes as a surprise to him and elicits a reaction of "Aha!"

The Threat

The mullah's donkey had been stolen. Full of rage, he ran to the bazaar and screamed with a loud voice, "Whoever took my donkey should bring him back immediately." Upset, with a red face and swollen veins in his neck, he continued shouting, "If I don't get my donkey back immediately, I'll do something I shouldn't do." The people standing around were visibly frightened by all this, but suddenly—no one knew who had brought it—the donkey was standing there. The crowd scattered. Everyone was happy that the problem had been resolved so smoothly. But an old man turned to the mullah and asked, "Tell me, what would you have done that you shouldn't do, if you hadn't gotten the donkey back?" The mullah answered, "What would I have done? I'd have bought another donkey, and you tell me if that would have been a wise thing to do with the thin money pouch I have."

The first part of this story encourages identification. Through the theft of his donkey, the mullah has become the victim of an injustice. He reacts with aggression and fantasies of omnipotence. "Something terrible will happen if . . ." On the basis of our own ideas about justice, it is easy for us to understand and endorse the mullah's threats.

But, at the same time, we know that a terrible event can produce unpleasant results, results which we can foresee in our mind's eye. This leads to a tension, which the mullah resolves in an

33

unexpected way, putting the situation in a new light. His demands for justice suddenly pale behind the motive of frugality. A new donkey would simply cost too much. The terrible event turns out not to be outwardly directed aggression. Instead, it is the conflict between the standards of frugality and the mullah's actual financial standing. This change of reference lessens the tension that has built up. Relieved, we react with a grin or chuckle. We can distance ourselves from the threatening situation. This process of displacement occurs with many stories. A change of perspective is suggested to the reader or listener. This new perspective has to do with the basic concepts.

Counter-concepts, as presented in stories, encourage changes in perspective and experimentation with unusual concepts and possible solutions. But, in this process, the central issue is not that the patient be led to retract the point of view he continues to hold despite many skirmishes. There's something else involved in the change of perspective: Familiar situations are seen from a new angle and thus are given a different character. Occasionally more change in perspective is all that is needed to solve the problem.

8.

Guidelines for the Reader

The Right Price

When King Anoschirwan traveled through the land with his people, he came to a desolate area in the mountains where there weren't even any pathetic little shepherd huts. The king's cook lamented, "Noble sultan! I am here to please your gums. But in our canteen we don't even have the littlest grain of salt. And without salt the food tastes terrible. Noble sultan, what should I do?" Anoschirwan replied, "Go back to the nearest town. There you'll find a merchant who has salt to sell. But be careful to pay the right price and not a bit more than is usual." "Noble sultan," answered the cook, "in your chest you have more money than anyone else in the world. What difference would it make to you if I pay a bit more for salt. That little bit won't amount to much." The king looked at him seriously and answered, "It is precisely the little things that grow into the injustices of the world. Little things are like drops of water that eventually fill an entire lake. The great injustices of the world began as little things. So go and buy the salt at the usual price."

Almost all the stories in this book are related to case examples, descriptions of real-life situations, and problems in interpersonal relations. The case presentations are examples and events that have taken place in my therapy practice or in connection with it. These cases reflect the uniqueness of the particular situation. They represent only one possible application of the story under consideration. This means that the steps taken to help one patient understand his conflict will not necessarily be successful for all seemingly similar cases

They should, however, stimulate the patient to more easily perceive human interactions and to be more sensitive to misunderstandings and their causes.

Each person can read the stories and interpret them for himself and his situation. They are didactic pieces that work without someone standing there with a raised finger; they are entertainment that does more than just entertain; they are guidelines, which each person can accept according to his needs. Just as we chose case examples from therapeutic practice, so each reader can infuse the stories with his own meaning, think about their message, and talk about them with other people. This is why I have not included interpretations for some of the stories in the final part of the book. They can stimulate the reader to continue in his own way what we have begun here.

The use of stories in Positive Psychotherapy is not arbitrary or coincidental. They are consciously positioned in the framework of the five-phase treatment and require on the part of the therapist sensitivity and insight into the patient's needs and the therapist's own motives. They also require the courage to give up the seemingly clearly structured form of the relationship and the courage to enter into fantasy and intuitive needs.

9.

Sources of the Stories

About the Difference between City Gates and Mouths

There once lived an Eastern king whose wisdom illuminated the land like a sun, whose cleverness was surpassed by no one, and whose wealth far exceeded that of everyone else. One day a vizier came to him with an unhappy face. "Great sultan, you are the wisest, greatest, and mightiest man in our land," he said. "You are lord over life and death. But what did I hear as I was traveling through the land? Everywhere the people praise you. But some people spoke very badly of you. They made jokes and complained about your wise decisions. How does it happen, you most mighty of all the mighty, that such insubordination exists in your realm?" The sultan smiled indulgently and answered, "Like every man in my kingdom, you know what I have accomplished for all of you. Seven lands are under my control. Under my rule, seven lands have achieved progress and prosperity. In seven lands, people love me because of my justice. You are certainly right. I can do many things. I can have the gigantic gates of my cities closed. But there is one thing I can't do. I cannot shut the mouths of my subjects. It is not really a question of what some people say bad about me. What is important is that I do good."

Some of the stories in this book are from classical Eastern literature and were adopted by such poets as Hafis, Saadi, Mowlana,

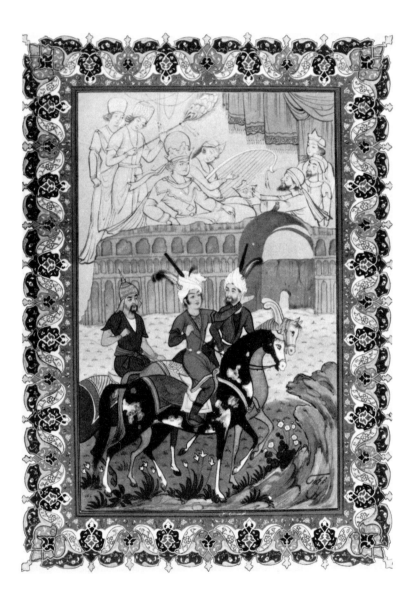

Parwin Etessami, and so forth (cf. biographical sketches, p. 157). To some extent, these stories have become known in the West through medical histories, Eastern studies, and literary works. Other stories are from folklore. They are transmitted orally, but until now hardly anyone bothered to write them down, let alone apply them to psychotherapy or social criticism. Then again, some stories are well known in the West in a similar form. People in the West regard them as anecdotes or jokes without knowing why they are told or why people laugh at them or wonder about them.

10.

The Favorite Character in Mideastern Literature

The Crow and the Parrot

A parrot was sitting with a crow in a cage. Ah, how the poor parrot suffered from the presence of the black-feathered monster! "What an ugly black, what a terrible figure, what an ordinary facial expression. If a person had to look at something like that at sunrise, his whole day would be ruined. There isn't a more disgusting companion than you anywhere."

As strange as it may seem, the crow also suffered from the presence of the parrot. Sad and depressed, the crow quarreled with the stroke of fate that had brought it together with that unpleasant multi-colored comrade. "Why does this bad luck have to strike me? Why did my lucky star forsake me? Why did my happy days end up in such days of darkness? It would have been much more pleasant to sit on a garden wall with another crow, enjoy the things we have in common, and to be happy."

(After Saadi)

Many stories take place at the level of caricature, thereby making it less painful for the listener to identify with the characters and their fates. This also enables the listener to maintain a sense of superiority. The hero's essential traits are lifted out and directed toward the point of the story. Other charateristics are simply disregarded. Aside from helping a person understand the story, this one-sidedness is also essential for the point of the story. Without

40

this imbalance and differentiation, the point would lose its effect as a surprise. From the perspective of narrowmindedness, the close connection between neurotic imbalance and the stories becomes clear. Put into general terms: We all have the potential to become comic figures for other people, namely when we produce narrowmindedness against the background of the relative values accepted by our sociocultural system.

The prototype of the "hero" in many Eastern stories is the *mullah*. He was a folk preacher who usually traveled through the country with his donkey. Since some very eccentric wandering preachers aroused the interest of the public and attracted attention with their jokes, irony, and clumsy behavior, the mullah became a popular figure in Persian folklore. Many things that could not be said openly because they would violate good manners, decorum, and tact were put into the mouth of the mullah or appeared in stories where he played a central role. For the Iranian people, the mullah had a function similar to that of the court jester in the courtly society of medieval Europe. As a caricature, he presented truth and wisdom, often in exaggerated ways, and carried them beyond the medium of story and joke. There are historical models for this process. Eight hundred years ago, the famous poet and social critic *Bahlull,* a close relative of the legendary caliph *Harun al Raschid,* let himself be declared insane. Thus safe from prosecution, he was able to go about under the fool's cap, helping to educate the populace.

As conveyor of the joke and as epitome of narrowmindedness, the mullah becomes a part of the individual ego. One can ascribe to him what one experiences in himself and dissociated parts of the personality. By so doing, he reestablishes inner harmony: It isn't I who expresses these irrational things, but the mullah in me. By naming him, I protect myself from threatening contents of my own self.

Through changes in perspective and the shift in concepts, the listener is forced to approach these strange, seemingly threatening, or at least ambivalent concepts—on an experimental basis, at least. In so doing, he expands his own concept on the level of feelings and the processing of experience. Procedures like this are thus appropriate as an entry into a therapeutic change of attitude or conduct.

41

11.

Self-Discovery

The Perfect Camel

Years ago four scholars traveled through the Kawir desert with a caravan. In the evening they sat together at the fire and talked about their experiences. They were all filled with admiration for the camels. They were amazed by their contentment, they admired their strength, and they found their modest patience to be almost incomprehensible. "We are the masters of the pen," the one said. "Let's write or draw about this animal this way to praise and honor the camel." As he said these words, he took a roll of parchment and went into a tent that was lit by an oil lamp. After a few minutes, he came out and showed his work to his three friends. He had drawn a camel just getting up from a resting position. The camel was so well drawn that one would almost think it were alive. The next man then went into the tent and soon came out. He brought a short factual depiction of the advantages that camels bring to a caravan. The third wrote an enchanting poem. Then a fourth man finally went into the tent and forbade the others to disturb him. A few hours later, the fire had gone out, and the others were already asleep. But, from the dimly lit tent, there still came the sound of the scratching of the pen and the monotonous song. The next day, the three waited just as futilely as they'd waited for their colleague on the second and third days. Like the cliffs that had closed behind Aladin, the tent hid the fourth scholar. Finally, on the fifth day, the entrance to the tent

42

opened up, and the most industrious of the industrious stepped out, dead tired, with black-rimmed eyes and sunken cheeks. His chin was framed by a stubbly beard. With tired steps and a look on his face as if he had eaten green lemons, he approached the other men. He wearily threw a bundle of parchments onto the carpet. On the outside of the first roll he had written in large letters, "The perfect camel, or how a camel should be . . ."

Like many other things, we have also learned our relationships to stories, fables and fairy tales. We have learned to love or reject them, or to react indifferently. There are some questions that can help us understand the sources of our attitudes toward stories:

Who read or told stories to you (father, mother, siblings, grandparents, aunt, kindergarten teacher, and so forth)?
Can you remember situations when stories were told to you?
How did you feel?
What do you think of fairy tales and stories?
Which story, narrative, or fairy tale comes to your mind automatically?
Who is your favorite author?
Which proverbs or concepts have the greatest significance for you?

For many people, it isn't fairy tales and fables that imprinted their relationship to stories. Rather, they associate them with religious parables and Bible stories. Some developed a preference for the imagery of the stories, but others acquired a deeply rooted distrust or emotional antipathy. But this response is sometimes more a reaction against the religious connection than against the stories per se.

Some examples for the meaning of religious parables appear in the first segment of Part II.

Part II

The Stories in Practice

1.

Parables

If I speak in the tongues of men and of angels, but have
not love, I am a noisy gong or a clanging cymbal.
(I Corinthians 13: 1)

Believe in God and Tie Your Camel Securely

*The faithful came in throngs to hear the words of the Prophet
Mohammed. One man listened especially attentively and devoutly, prayed
with faith and fervor, and finally left the prophet when evening came. He
was hardly outside when he came running back in and cried out with an
excited voice, "O my lord! This morning I rode my camel to hear you, the
prophet of God. Now the camel is gone. Far and wide, there's not a camel
in sight. I was obedient to you, heeded your every word, and trusted in
God's power. Now, O lord, my camel is gone. Is that divine justice? Is that
the reward for my faith? Is that the thanks for my prayers?" Mohammed
listened to these desperate words and answered with a kindly smile, "Believe
in God and tie your camel securely."*

The language of religions is a language in images. Almost all
religious texts avoid proclaiming commandments and prohibitions
in straightforward language; they can't be compared to our books of
law, where the language is plain and nuance is sacrificed for

47

precision. It makes no difference whether the proclaimer himself uses similes, parables, and verbal images in the religious texts, or whether the life of the proclaimer is presented as a model; everywhere we find stylistic devices that are similar to those in stories, fables and mythologies.

Stories seem to be suitable transmitters of moral, philosophic, and religious messages. Even in religious parables, models are presented for emulation or to serve as a deterrent. They give the believer concrete information about how he should act as a member of his religious community; they show which models he should use as a guide. In conjunction with the Koran, the following is a story about Ali, Mohammed's son-in-law.

The Date-Eater

A woman came with her little boy to the wise Ali and said, "My son is suffering from a serious problem. He eats dates from morning till night. If I don't give him any dates, he screams his head off. What shall I do? Please help me." The wise Ali looked at the child kindly and said, "My good woman, go home and come back at the same time tomorrow." The next day, the woman and her son again stood before Ali. The great master sat the boy on his lap, spoke to him in a friendly way and finally took the dates out of his hand as he said, "My son, think always of moderation. There are other things that taste good." With these words, he let the mother and child go. The woman, who was somewhat puzzled, asked "Great master, why didn't you say that yesterday? Why did we have to make the long trip to you a second time?" "My good lady," Ali answered, "yesterday I couldn't have convincingly told your son what I told him today, because yesterday I myself had savored the sweetness of the dates."

Almost all religions have experienced a turn toward specialization. The rabbis were the transmitters of the Old Testament teachings; the church fathers and Roman Catholic popes became the teachers of the New Testament. In Islam, the imams and, on a lower level, the mullah (Akhunden) conveyed religious contents.

But, on the other hand, the holy scriptures of these religions emphasize that an understanding of their teachings is not reserved only for a few scholars; no one is "more equal" than the rest. By means of various parables,these writings all imply that everyone can come to terms with religious contents. Christ used the child as a symbol of the person who can come close to religious truth by himself and without a lot of sophistry.

The following story is told about a Bábi, a disciple of Báb (forerunner of the Bahá'i religion):

The Scholar and the Camel Driver

In a caravan crossing the desert, there was once a learned preacher who was so wise that he brought along seventy camels, each loaded with heavy chests. In them there was nothing but the scholar's books about the wisdoms of the past and present. This load of books was only a drop in the bucket compared to the knowledge the preacher carried around in his head.

Accompanying the caravan was a poor camel driver of whom it was known that he believed the last imman (the new prophet) had come. It had to happen, of course, that the preacher one day summoned the camel driver. "You know how famous I am among the scholars of the country and the whole world," he said. "You see the seventy camels that carry only a fraction of my knowledge. How does it happen that you, a simple camel driver in ragged clothes, who has never even learned to read and write, who didn't even attend a school, let alone an academy, can dare believe the last imman has come?"

The camel driver stood modestly in front of the elegant gentleman, bowed politely, and said, "Effendi, my lord. I would never have dared to step before you and direct my meager words to you. But now you've asked me. I'll try to show you what I think by giving a little example. Lord! You have control of a wonderful treasury of knowledge, which I would like to compare to the finest pearls in the sea. These pearls are so valuable that they have to be kept in an exquisitely decorated chest, wrapped in soft, velvet cloths. Compared to all this, my knowledge is like the ordinary stones we step on in the desert. But imagine the sun coming up. It sends its rays to us. My lord, here is my question for you: What catches the sun's rays and reflects their glow? Your precious pearls in their prison of velvet, or my pathetic stones on the side of the road?"

49

Whether they belong to the Holy Scriptures or whether they are told and transmitted in connection with them, stories serve to elucidate the religious concepts of the prophets. Moses' ten commandments, which are equally valid in Judaism and Christianity, in Islam and in the Bahá'i religion, are exemplified and made comprehensible by stories. They are carried beyond the abstract level of commandments—"Thou shalt not . . ."—into the real world of the faithful. Here there are also pedagogical realizations as they relate to the concepts of religion. The following tale about Ali, Mohammed's son-in-law, is to a certain extent an illustration of the commandment "Thou shalt not steal." It can also be used as an introduction for treating people who have broken this commandment or are in a position to violate the standard norms and proscriptions of their group.

The Truthful Thief

To an honorable wise man, there was once brought a young thief who had been caught stealing. But, because of his youth, they didn't want to punish him as severely as the law required. The wise man was supposed to show the boy the dismal path and the wretched end of a life of thievery, and thereby break him of this disgusting practice. But the wise man didn't say a word about stealing. He spoke kindly to the boy and won his trust. The only demand he made was that the boy promise always to be truthful. Thinking he'd really gotten off easily, the boy readily agreed to this and went home feeling very relieved. But, during the night, thoughts about stealing came to him in the same way that clouds darken the moon. As he crept through a side door of his house, however, he was struck by a thought: "What will I say if someone stops me on the street and asks what I'm doing? What will I say tomorrow? If I keep my promise to be truthful, I have to confess everything and can't avoid the punishment I deserve." As the boy tried to be truthful despite all his habits, it became hard for him to steal. The development of his truthfulness provided space for his honesty and justness.

The Proper Prayer

While on a trip, Abdu'l-Bahá, the son of Bahá'u'lláh, the founder of the Bahá'i religion, had been invited to dinner with a family. The wife had good intentions and wanted to show her great culinary artistry. When she brought out the food, she apologized for the fact that it was burned. While cooking it, she had been reading prayers in the hope that the meal would be especially successful. 'Abdu'l-Bahá answered with a friendly smile and said, "It's good that you pray. But next time you're in the kitchen, pray from a cookbook."

This story illustrates the close ties between religion and daily life, which the devout adherent of a religion clearly perceives. It deals with the difference between religious and everyday tasks and aptly points out religious narrowmindedness and the mental disorders that stem from the confrontation with ecclesiastical rules of morality.

The Pharisee and the Publican

Jesus told this parable to some who trusted in themselves that they were righteous and despised others:

Two men went up into the temple to pray, one a Pharisee and the other a tax collector. The Pharisee stood and prayed thus with himself, "God, I thank thee that I am not like other men, extortionists, unjust, adulterers, or even like this tax collector. I fast twice a week, I give tithes of all that I get." But the tax collector, standing far off, would not even lift up his eyes to heaven, but beat his breast, saying "God, be merciful to me, a sinner!" I tell you, this man went down to his house justified rather than the other; for everyone who exalts himself will be humbled, but he who humbles himself will be exalted.

(Luke 18: 9–14)

This story was used directly as a parable or didactic piece. Genres of this nature appear in great numbers in the New Testament. After posing a question about a concrete situation, the disciples and listeners are confronted with a story as a parable. These parables were taken from daily events of that period and use characters whose role and significance was clear at that time. An example of this is the publican, who was both tax collector and constable.

The Log in Your Own Eye

Judge not, that you be not judged.

For with the judgment you pronounce you will be judged, and the measure you give will be the measure you get. Why do you see the speck that is in your brother's eye, but do not notice the log that is in your own eye? Or how can you say to your brother, "Let me take the speck out of your eye," when there is a log in your own eye? You hypocrite, first take the log out of your own eye, and then you will see clearly to take the speck out of your brother's eye.

(Matthew 7: 1–5)

Metaphors such as the ones in these verses have multiple meanings. Their image contains more than their words say. Along with its significance for the social and individual need for justice, the example of the log in one's eye is an excellent description of projection, the transference of one's own needs and feelings of guilt. These verses thus also contain the command that one first look at his own problems before he turn to the problems of his partner, fellow-man, or patients—whether in a therapeutic sense or in the role of judge.

The command that we first see the log in our own eye before seeing the speck in others' eyes corresponds in another sense to the professional ethics of the psychotherapist. In the course of his training he himself undergoes psychotherapy before he goes about treating patients.

The Sun-Crier

In the chicken yard, the rooster was so ill that no one could count on his crowing the next morning. The hens were very worried that the sun wouldn't rise if the crowing of their lord and master did not summon it. The hens, you see, thought the sun came up only because the rooster crowed. The next day the sun cured them of their superstition. To be sure, the rooster was still too sick and too hoarse to crow, but the sun shone anyway; nothing had affected its course.

(Persian Fairy Tale after 'Abdu'l-Bahá)

Man's relationship to God can be described only in simile and image. Even mathematical formulas to prove the existence of a spirit controlling the universe are, in the end, only similes. They attempt to come at least a few steps closer to the unkown and unrecognizable.

Shadows on the Sundial

In the East, a king once wanted to please his subjects. Since they did not know what a clock was, he brought back a sundial from one of his trips. His gift changed the lives of the people in the kingdom. They began to differentiate parts of the day and to divide up their time. Becoming more prompt, orderly, reliable, and industrious, they produced great wealth and a high standard of living. When the king died, his subjects wondered how they could pay tribute to his achievements. Because the sundial symbolized the king's generosity and was the cause for their success, they decided to build around it a splendid temple with a golden cupola. But, when the temple was finished and the cupola soared above the sundial, the rays of the sun no longer reached the dial. The shadow, which had told the time for the citizens had disappeared; the common point of orientation, the sundial, was covered. The one citizen was no longer punctual, the other no longer reliable, the third no longer industrious. Each went his own way. The kingdom collapsed.

This Eastern folktale takes up the simile of light. Light, which

53

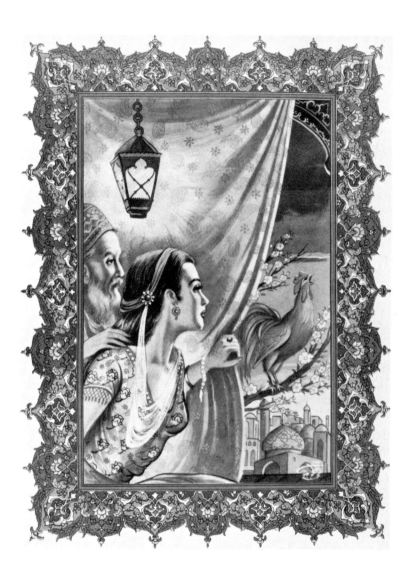

represents the essence of truth for the followers of Zarathustra, is placed in connection with human talents. In a different metaphor, the factors working against man's talents are compared to the dirt that darkens the surface of a mirror. But here they are rewritten as a temple. As the next example shows 'Abdu'l-Bahá has expanded the iridescent quality of human talents by stressing the concept of uniqueness. The teacher is compared to a gardener, and the human, the child, is like a plant.

The Teacher, a Gardener

"A teacher's work is like that of a gardener who takes care of various plants. One plant loves the sunshine, the other the cool shade; one loves the shore of the stream, the other the barren mountain peak. One thrives in sandy soil, the other in rich loam. Each requires the care best suited for it; otherwise the result is unsatisfactory."

(Abdu'l-Bahá)

This is an appropriate place for the description of the relationship between body and soul, as given by Bahá'u'lláh:

The Relationship between Soul and Body

"Know thou that the soul of man is exalted above, and is independent of all infirmities of body or mind. That a sick person showeth signs of weakness is due to the hindrances that interpose themselves between his soul and his body, for the soul itself remaineth unaffected by any bodily ailments. Consider the light of the lamp. Though an external object may interfere with its radiance, the light itself continueth to shine with undiminished power. In like manner, every malady afflicting the body of man is an impediment that preventeth the soul from manifesting its inherent might and power. When it leaveth the body, however, it will evince such ascendancy, and reveal such influence as no force on earth can equal. Every pure, every refined and sanctified soul will be endowed with tremendous power, and shall rejoice with exceeding gladness.

"Consider the lamp which is hidden under a bushel. Though its light be shining, yet its radiance is concealed from men. Likewise, consider the sun which hath been obscured by the clouds. Observe how its splendor appeareth to have diminished, when in the reality the source of that light hath remained unchanged. The soul of man should be likened unto this sun, and all things on earth should be regarded as his body. So long as no external impediment interveneth between them, the body will, in its entirety, continue to reflect the light of the soul, and to be sustained by its power. As soon as, however, a veil interposeth itself between them, the brightness of that light seemeth to lessen.

"Consider again the sun when it is completely hidden behind the clouds. Though the earth is still illumined with its light, yet the measure of light which it receiveth is considerably reduced. Not until the clouds have dispersed, can the sun shine again in the plenitude of its glory. Neither the presence of the cloud nor its absence can, in any way, affect the inherent splendor of the sun. The soul of man is the sun by which his body is illumined, and from which it draweth its sustenance, and should be so regarded.

"Consider, moreover, how the fruit, ere it is formed, lieth potentially within the tree. Were the tree to be cut into pieces, no sign nor any part of the fruit, however small, could be detected. When it appeareth, however, it manifesteth itself, as thou hast observed, in its wondrous beauty and glorious perfection. Certain fruits, indeed, attain their fullest development only after being severed from the tree."

(Gleanings from the Writings of Bahá'u'lláh, p. 153 ff.)

Crisis as Opportunity

"There was once a lover who had sighed for long years in separation from his beloved, and wasted in the fire of remoteness. From the rule of love, his heart was empty of patience, and his body weary of his spirit; he reckoned life without her as a mockery, and time consumed him away. How many a day he found no rest in longing for her; how many a night the pain of her kept him from sleep; his body was worn to a sigh, his heart's wound had turned him to a cry of sorrow. He had given a thousand lives for one taste of the cup of her presence, but it availed him not. The doctors knew no

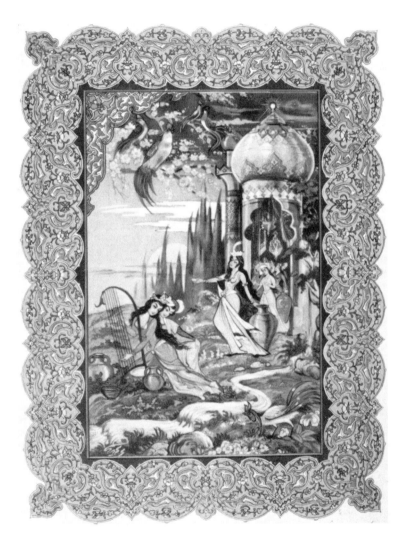

cure for him, and companions avoided his company; yea, physicians have no medicine for one sick of love, unless the favor of the beloved one deliver him.

"At last, the tree of his longing yielded the fruit of despair, and the fire of his hope fell to ashes. Then one night he could live no more, and he went out of his house and made for the market-place. On a sudden, a watchman followed after him. He broke into a run, with the watchman following; then other watchmen came together, and barred every passage to the weary one. And the wretched one cried from his heart, and ran here and there, and moaned to himself: 'Surely this watchman is Izrá'íl, my angel of death, following so fast upon me; or he is a tyrant of men, seeking to harm me.' His feet carried him on, the one bleeding with the arrow of love, and his heart lamented. Then he came to a garden wall, and with untold pain he scaled it, for it proved very high; and forgetting his life, he threw himself down to the garden.

"And there he beheld his beloved with a lamp in her hand, searching for a ring she had lost. When the heart-surrendered lover looked on his ravishing love, he drew a great breath and raised up his hands in prayer, crying: 'O God! Give Thou glory to the watchman, and riches and long life. For the watchman was Gabriel, guiding this poor one; or he was Isráfíl, bringing life to this wretched one!'

"Indeed, his words were true, for he had found many a secret justice in this seeming tyranny of the watchman, and seen how many a mercy lay hid behind the veil. Out of wrath, the guard had led him who was athirst in love's desert to the sea of his loved one, and lit up the dark night of absence with the light of reunion. He had driven one who was afar, into the garden of nearness, had guided an ailing soul to the heart's physician.

"Now if the lover could have looked ahead, he would have blessed the watchman at the start, and prayed on his behalf, and he would have seen that tyranny as justice; but since the end was veiled to him, he moaned and made his plaint in the beginning. Yet those who journey in the garden-land of knowledge, because they see the end in the beginning, see peace in war and friendliness in anger.

"Such is the state of the wayfarers in this Valley; but the people of the Valleys above this see the end and the beginning as one; nay, they see neither beginning nor end, and witness neither 'first' nor 'last.'"

(Bahá'u'lláh, *Seven Valleys,* 1975, P. 14 ff.)

"The stages that mark the wayfarer's journey from the abode of dust to the heavenly homeland are said to be seven. Some have called these Seven Valleys, and others, Seven Cities. And they say that until the wayfarer taketh leave of self, and traverseth these stages, he shall never reach to the ocean of nearness and union, nor drink of the peerless wine."

(Bahá'u'lláh, *Seven Valleys* p.4)

Solomon's Judgment

Then two harlots came to the king, and stood before him. The one woman said, "Oh, my lord, this woman and I dwell in the same house; and I gave birth to a child while she was in the house. Then on the third day after I was delivered, this woman also gave birth; and we were alone; there was no one else with us in the house. And this woman's son died in the night, because she lay on it. And she arose at midnight, and took my son from beside me, while your maidservant slept, and laid it in her bosom, and laid her dead son in my bosom. When I rose in the morning to nurse my child, behold, it was dead; but when I looked at it closely in the morning, behold, it was not the child that I had borne."

But the other woman said, "No, the living child is mine, and the dead child is yours." The first said, "No, the dead child is yours and the living child is mine." Thus they spoke before the king. Then the king said, "The one says, 'This is my son that is alive, and your son is dead'; and the other says, 'No; but your son is dead, and my son is the living one.'" And the king said, "Bring me a sword." So a sword was brought before the king. And the king said, "Divide the living child in two, and give half to the one, and half to the other." Then the woman whose son was alive said to the king, because her heart yearned for her son, "Oh, my lord, give her the living child, and by no means slay it." But the other said, "It shall be neither mine nor yours; divide it." Then the king answered, "Give the living child to the first woman, and by no means slay it; she is its mother." And all Israel heard of the judgment which the king had rendered; and they stood in awe of the king, because they perceived that the wisdom of God was in him, to render justice.

(I Kings 3: 16–28)

The Old Testament as one of the Holy Scriptures of the Jews, seems at first glance to be more a genealogy of the forefathers of ancient Israel and an interesting history book. But along with descriptions of events, it contains images and parables that go beyond mere historical summary or the enumeration of moral and ethical commandments. Each of the accounted events is in some way important and instructive for people today; it can be effective in the sense of a folk psychotherapy. A good example of this is Solomon's judgment, which sounds very modern and could serve as precedent for divorce judgments and decisions on child custody. Not the one who demands strict pronouncements of justice, but the one who is willing to make sacrifices for the benefit of the child or partner, is qualified to bear the responsibility.

Bertolt Brecht took up the theme of Solomon's judgment in a modern version. But instead of using the feudal ruler Solomon as his mouthpiece, he used the clever judge Azdak. Brecht also did away with using a sword; he lets the two mothers fight for the child by trying to pull it to their respective sides.

What is only hinted at in Solomon's judgment, and was prevented by the goodness and motherly feelings of one of the quarreling parties, namely the splitting of the child, has often taken place—in the realm of divorce—in the experiences and feelings of children. They are heart and soul with their mothers, but driven by a sense of guilt or need for justice, stand up for their fathers. They are inwardly torn apart. These observations call forth a thought experiment. Solomon's judgment requires a maternal heart and the one woman's ability to renounce her claims. How would Solomon have reacted if, as we often see today, both parties demanded their rights without regard for the welfare of the one whom they are fighting for?

Justice in the Beyond

A mullah preached from his chancel, "Blessed are they who live in poverty. Whoever runs around on earth naked because he cannot buy clothes, will wear the most priceless fabrics in the next world." He turned to a poor man dressed in rags, who was staring at him with hungry eyes. "You, my good friend, are my neighbor. I say to you, in the next world you will be dressed in fabrics which you have never touched before, and you will eat foods you haven't even smelled from afar. But I say this to you under one condition: When I come to you in that other world and want something from you, don't forget that I was your neighbor."

The poor and unjustly treated person is given the prospect of justice in the next world. But even this is not free of self-interest. The hope which the Mullah kindles is like alms which are given to a beggar, not to help him, but to mollify one's own sense of guilt and responsibilities and to better secure one's own salvation. The Mullah does not offer a slice of bread or money so that the poor man can quiet his hunger. He gives only some words which promise hope.

What Distinguishes the Hakim from the Prophet?

Avicena was once approached by a student who respected him greatly. The man spoke, "Great master, you are wiser than the learned of our time. You are a philosopher, physician, poet, astrologer. You know all that, and even more than the science of our day requires. Why don't you proclaim that you are a prophet? I'm convinced that thousands and thousands will follow you and heed your words. You see, Mohammed was only a camel driver, inexperienced in the sciences, and yet his word reached the ears of millions."

"I will explain it to you when the time is right," answered Avicena. "Just be patient."

In the following winter, colder than even the oldest people could remember, Avicena was bedridden with illness. In the same room, there was also that student who had questioned him. It was night. Dried out from fever, Avicena was thirsty for a sip of cool water. "Friend," he said to his roommate, "I'm very thirsty. Would you bring me a glass of water from outside?"

At the thought of going out into the miserable cold, the student crawled further down into his covers. "No, master," he said, "the doctors all agree that, in your condition, cold water would be poison."

61

Avicena's thirst grew. His tongue lay dry in his mouth. "Go ahead and bring me some water. For my illness, something cool is the best remedy."

But the thought of having to break the ice at the well outside to fulfill his master's wish gave the companion a good case of gooseflesh. Unyielding, he continued to argue that there was nothing worse than cold water. But Avicena, the great physician, kept insisting that only cold water could relieve his suffering. The two men began a quarrel over dogma that eventually went on all night.

At dawn there rang forth from the tower of the minaret the voice of the muezzin, who summoned the faithful to cleanse themselves as the prophet commanded, to bow their heads toward Mecca, and to speak the holy Suren. Avicena's pupil threw his blanket aside, jumped out of bed, stormed out of the room, cracked the ice on the well and bathed as his faith prescribed. Then he knelt down on the prayer rug to offer the morning prayer, a song of praise.

After he had finished his prayers, Avicena spoke to him. "Dear friend, you still remember asking me why I don't claim to be a prophet. Today I want to answer you. See, Mohammed, who was only a camel driver, has already been gone from us over three-hundred years, and yet his word has the power and might to get you out of a warm bed; it has the power to cause you to bathe with cold ice water and say your prayers in spite of the cold. When I begged you all night to get me a glass of water, all my words were still too weak, although I know that you revere me as your master. This is one of the reasons why, despite my learnedness, I will never claim to be a prophet."

Above all else, this story makes one thing clear: Regardless of how trusting the patient is, the therapist can hardly fall back on the charisma which belongs only to a prophet.

2.

Physicians' Perplexity and Hope

The Miracle of the Ruby

A sheik announced in the coffeehouse that the caliph had forbidden singing. When a dervish heard this, he was so sad that his innermost being shrunk together into a lump, and a severe illness took possession of him. The experienced hakim was called to his sickbed. He felt his pulse and examined him according to the rules of his art, but he could not bring the illness into harmony with what he had read in the great books of medicine, and not even with the experiences of his many years of medical practice.

The dervish breathed his last breath, and the hakim, thirsty for knowledge, cut open the corpse. There, where the dervish had felt the greatest pain, he found a large lump as red as a ruby. Later on when financial problems troubled him, the hakim sold the stone. It then passed from hand to hand until it finally came into the possession of the caliph. He had it set in a ring.

One day, as he was wearing the ring again, the caliph began to sing. At the same moment his robe turned blood red, without his body having a single wound. Astonished, he watched how his ruby bubbled up like hot oil and spread over his robe like blood. Shocked by this miracle, he wanted to trace the secret of the ruby. He summoned its previous owners, one by one, until he reached the hakim. The hakim was now able to explain the mystery to him.

(After Mowlana)

Although the ancient Eastern physician was oriented toward the wealthy classes, his role had at the same time a charitable meaning linked to religious precepts. In many medical offices, the sign was posted announcing "Thursday afternoon (the day before the holy Friday), needy patients are treated free." This saying can still be found today in some centers that adhere to tradition.

The hakim combined a number of roles and tasks in one person. His practice was far less specialized than that of today's doctor. It comprised diagnostic measures like urine tests, pulse checks, and careful examination of the patient, as well as therapeutic conversation and measures that remind one of contemporary psychosomatic medicine.

Poets and storytellers of ancient Persia told of the activity of favored doctors and ridiculed the charlatanry of the quacks. Of course, the good, experienced doctor was more accessible to the nobility and the rich. But, through a series of stories and writings similar to didactic literature, they supplied a report; even those who could not afford them could still benefit from the wisdom of the hakim and draw lessons from it, without having to pay a fee.

To understand these stories, it is necessary to consider the situation prevailing at that time. Sultan, king, ruler, and sheik exercised feudal rule. To be sure, the doctor was highly regarded, but provided service in the same way as did a courtier, soldier, or governor. Along with that, the doctor was somewhat like a merchant who moved from place to place and offered his wares or skills for sale. In addition, it was his job to harmonize the patient's pain with the religious principles, and to establish connections with revealed wisdom. The possible indignation against Allah (God) because of ostensible injustice was thus intercepted by the physician.

The Shared Sorrows

"Go on and sleep; tomorrow is also a day from God," groaned a wife, after her husband had tossed and turned a hundred times. "When you are so restless, I can't sleep either." "Ah, wife," complained the husband, "if you

had my problems. A few months ago, I signed a note, and tomorrow it's due. Poor me! You know I don't have a bit of money in the house, and you also know that our neighbor, to whom I owe the money, can be more poisonous than a scorpion when it's a question of money. Poor me! How could I sleep?" At that point, he again tossed back and forth ten times. All his wife's attempts to calm him down and to strew the sands of sleep in his eyes were to no avail. She tried to comfort him by saying, "Wait till morning: then things will look different, and perhaps we'll find a way to pay the money." "Nothing, nothing will work," groaned the man. "Everything is lost." Finally his wife lost her patience. She went out onto the roof garden and called over to the neighbor, "You know, my husband owes you a debt which comes due tomorrow. I want to tell you something you don't know. My husband can't pay the debt tomorrow." Without waiting for an answer the woman ran back into the bedroom and said, "If I can't sleep, my neighbor shouldn't either." Full of defiance, she crawled into bed while her husband pulled the sheet high up over his ears and lay there anxiously, his teeth chattering. Soon all was quiet, and nothing more could be heard but the even breathing of the couple.

(Persian Story)

Folk psychotherapy not conducted by doctors uses methods characterized most of all by craftiness and cunning. One tried, as well as one could, to outdo one's partner, opponent, the prevailing norms and social force, and even one's own fears. In so doing, there are many kinds of relief, one of which is described in the story of the shared sorrows. The wife helped herself and her husband by establishing justice as she understood it: If I can't sleep because of my problems, why should the other person? This subjective justice, of course, does not solve the problem. The debts are not paid off in this way, but one has the feeling of not being helplessly handed over to the one holding the note. The one with the note is now no better off than the debtor himself.

The Magician

The mullah, a preacher, wanted to get some nuts for his wife, because she had promised to cook him fesenjan, a dish prepared with nuts. In the joy

65

of anticipating his favorite dish, the mullah reached deep into the nut jar and grabbed as many nuts as he could reach with one hand. When he tried to pull his arm out of the jar, it was stuck. As hard as he pulled and twisted, the jar would not release his arm. He cried, groaned, and cursed as a mullah really shouldn't. But nothing helped. Even when his wife took the jar and pulled on it with all her weight, nothing happened. His hand remained stuck in the neck of the jar. After many futile attempts, they called their neighbors for help. Everyone followed with great interest this play which was going on in front of them. One of the neighbors took a look at the problem and asked the mullah how this accident had happened. With a pathetic voice and moans of desperation, the mullah told of the mishap. His neighbor said, "I will help you if you do exactly as I say."

"I promise to do everything you say, if you can just free me from this terrible jar."

"Then shove your arm farther into the jar."

This seemed strange to the mullah, for why should he put his arm farther into the jar when he wanted to get it out of there? But he did as he was told.

The neighbor continued, "Now open your hand, and drop the nuts you are holding." This request upset the mullah. After all, he wanted the nuts for his favorite dish, and now he was supposed just to drop them. Reluctantly, he followed his helper's directions. The man now said, "Make your hand very small, and pull it slowly out of the jar."

The mullah did this, and, behold, without any truble, he pulled his hand out of the jar. But he wasn't completely satisfied. "My hand is free now, but where are the nuts?" At that the neighbor took the jar, tipped it over, and let as many nuts roll out as the mullah needed. Wide-eyed and with open mouth, the mullah watched and said, "Are you a magician?"

(Persian Story)

Much has changed in psychotherapy since the days of psychotherapeutic practice in the ancient East. Familiarity with inner problems and disturbed behavior has been increasingly systematized and put into scientific connections. The functions of learning were differentiated; the dynamics of the personality and its intrinsicalness in the social context were discovered. But, in one respect at least, the role of the therapist has not changed essentially.

Then as today, he carries with him the image of a magician who can control the mysterious, the supernatural and the mystic; he can lend clarity to the dark side of the soul, just as the X ray pierces the human body. As flattering as this view may be for the therapist, it becomes a hindrance in the therapeutic process; disappointments arise when recovery does not occur immediately. Therapeutically, of course, such a reaction can be understood and handled as a defense mechanism, resistance, or the need for an almighty "Father." Nevertheless, the magician-therapist, as he is represented in the consciousness of many potential patients, is a problem for psychotherapy and its image with the public.

The Wish Dream

To the hakim there came a white-haired, toothless sheik who complained, "You helper of mankind, help me, too. I barely fall asleep, and a dream gets control of me. I dream I am coming to the front plaza of a harem. Women are there like the flowers of a garden, the apples of a tree, and the houris of paradise. I barely enter the court, and they disappear into a secret corridor."

The hakim wrinkled his brow, thought very carefully about it, and finally asked, "You probably want me to give you some powder or a medicine to ward against this dream."

Flabbergasted, the sheik cried out, "No, not that. The only thing I want is that, in the dream, the door to the secret passage be locked so that the women cannot run away from me.

Children would say, "A dream is movies in your sleep." There is a lot of truth in this simple definition. In a dream, actions run their course, and experiences and events occur in a way that leaves the dreamer wondering if he is the hero of the dream or merely a spectator. Physiology attributes dreams to a stage of sleep. There are various opinions about what dreams mean: predictions of the future, the processing of experience, the language of the unconscious. This last view has been a major concern of psychoanalysis, which proceeds from the following considerations: contents, suppressed and pushed aside in the waking hours, disguise themselves as symbols during sleep, a period of less control. These symbols direct the interpreter to the contents they represent. In the dream language of symbolism, there appear before the eyes of the dreamer actions, figures, and stories that are sometimes conscious only for the duration of the dream and are then forgotten again—or they can occupy a person for hours, days, or even a lifetime.

The meaning of these dream stories is rarely clear or unequivocal; it depends directly on the interpretations and one's understanding of them. Just as we tell each other stories in social situations, so we tell ourselves stories in our dreams. But we do not at first know their origin or outcome. It is as if another person were telling us things to which we react strongly. We empathize and rejoice accordingly. Perhaps, in the dream, our fantasy, as a medium and as a place of resolution, takes on the significance denied it in our rationally determined daily life. Dreams are thus stories linked closely to personality; they are individual mythologies that reflect reality in their own way and give us entry to a completely personal understanding of reality.

Psychoanalysis and depth psychology call the dream the king's path *(via regia)* to the unconscious. This realization can be employed therapeutically inasmuch as the patient takes on the task of discussing his dreams and associating with them, and the therapist supports him in this process by explaining the dreams.

The dream works as a therapeutic medium that is inserted into the relationship between therapist and patient. It deals primarily with the individual's own history. There is a similar function in the transmitted stories of cultures and groups. But in these cases they deal with the collective past of those groups. It is therefore hard to draw a line between dream and story, between individual and collective mythology. One reason for this is that many things that play a role in the life of a culture or group are also involved in an individual's processing of his experiences. And second, the members of a group repeatedly employ similar and comparable themes and motives for their collective tradition.

Whom Should You Believe?

"Can you lend me your donkey for this afternoon?" a farmer asked the mullah.

"Dear friend," replied the mullah, "you know that I am always ready to give you help when you need it. My heart longs to lend my donkey to you, an orthodox man. It pleases my eye to see you bring home the fruits of the field with my donkey. But what can I say, my dear friend? At the moment, someone else has my donkey."

Moved by the mullah's sincerity, the farmer thanked him profusely by saying, "Well, even if you couldn't help me, your kind words have helped me a great deal. May God be with you, O noble, kind, and wise mullah." But, as the farmer was still frozen in a deep bow, there came from the stall a bloodcurdling heehaw. The farmer was startled, looked up in astonishment, and finally asked mistrustingly, "What do I hear? Your donkey is there after all. I heard his donkeylike voice."

The mullah turned red with anger and screamed, "You ungrateful man. I told you the donkey is not there. Whom do you believe more: the mullah or the stupid cries of an even more stupid donkey?"

Many people, physicians as well as patients, wear blinders. They believe that only certain causes of illnesses can be proven. Other possible reasons and backgrounds for sickness are disregarded. For a long time, psychosomatics was also outside the general field of vision. This narrowing of perspective was encouraged by the fantastic successes in somatic medicine. Evident connections between social, mental, and physical realms were overlooked. Problems in the workplace, abnormal mourning after the death of a loved one, continued difficulties within the family were unacceptable as causes for illness. Only the physical symptoms were treated and, with the introduction of appropriate medication, the mental symptoms. On the other hand, we find dogmatic convictions that go in the opposite direction. In order not to falsify the psychotherapy, and to prevent the transference of mental problems, some people completely avoid all medication, even when it could mean a decrease in the unbearable suffering the patient endures.

69

It seems important to see and listen carefully to each case and test its conditions before choosing one or the other approach, or a combination of the two. Deciding whom to believe is, to a great extent, left to the patient, for he has the right to be informed about his illness and to find out the meaning of the therapeutic measures. For these reasons it seems important to us that doctors not necessarily schooled in psychotherapy know of the potentials and limits of psychotherapy, so they can lead their patients to the most appropriate therapy as soon as possible. This requirement is all the more urgent when we keep in mind that it takes almost six years for a patient with psychosomatic disorders, hence physical illnesses linked to mental causes, to locate a specialist in psychotherapy.

Limiting oneself to therapeutic treatment eventually comes into conflict with the patient's desire to have an "all powerful" doctor. Along with the trust that patients have in their doctor, there is today also the expectation that the doctor knows everything; the patient likes to interpret it as a sign of weakness if the doctor admits his professional limitations. More than a few patients or their loved ones want a physician like the one in the following story.

The Hakim Knows Everything

A man lay bedridden with a serious illness, and it appeared that his death was near. In her fear, his wife summoned a hakim, the town doctor. The hakim tapped around on the patient and listened for more than a half hour, checked his pulse, put his head on the man's chest, turned him onto his stomach and then his side and back, raised the man's legs and torso, opened his eyes, looked in his mouth, and then said with a great deal of conviction, "My dear woman, unfortunately I must give you the sad news that your husband has been dead for two days." At this very moment the ailing man raised his head in shock and whimpered anxiously, "No, my dearest, I'm still alive." The wife gave her husband a hefty slap on the head with her fist and replied angrily, "Be quiet! The hakim, a doctor, is an expert. He ought to know."

(Persian Story)

The patient has the potential for illness and for health. The therapist takes over a function that regulates the patient's illness and health. He can influence the patient's receptiveness to illness, but can also mobilize and stabilize his potential for health. This task is the dominant goal of preventive medicine and psycho-hygiene.

Treatment in Roundabout Ways

As court physician for the ruler Nuhe-Samani, Avicena took part in a celebration at the court. A lady of the court brought out a large fruit bowl. As she bowed down to hand Avicena a piece of fruit, she was unable to straighten up again and screamed with pain. She had been stricken by lumbago. The ruler looked at Avicena sternly and ordered him to help her. Avicena thought a moment as he panicked inwardly. He had left all his medicines at home and would have to seek new remedies. With this in mind, he grabbed into the woman's blouse. She pulled back horrified and then shrieked because of the pains which were now even worse. The king was enraged by Avicena's impudent behavior. But before he could say something, the doctor nimbly grabbed under the lady's skirt and tried to pull down her underwear. The girl blushed with embarrassment and defended herself by jumping out of the way. As if by a miracle, her pains disappeared. She straightened up easily without any pain. Satisfied, Avicena rubbed his hands and said, "Very good. Even she could be helped."

In spite of—or perhaps because of—technical and theoretical deficiencies, the procedures of the old hakims were often ingenious. Aside from the humor in this story, Avicena's action is instructive.

Let's assume he knew that a lumbago patient's discomfort is simply increased by the imbalanced posture the patient adopts because of fear of further pain. In this case he would have had the opportunity to relax the cramping by using a method used, for example, in chiropractic or physical therapy. The situation was urgent, however, and, as a hakim, he was also an artist from whom the king demanded an immediate proof of his art. He therefore took a different approach.

71

Figuring the woman would be embarrassed in front of all those people if he attacked her sexually, he developed his strategy. In the back of his mind, he seems to have had the idea that modesty, the fear of being revealed in front of other people, and, along with this, the sexual taboo, were stronger than fear of severe pain, which kept her immobile. As the story shows, Avicena's calculations were correct. His procedure, using psycho-social norms to effect conduct and, hence, the body, is an example of social-psychosomatic treatment.

The Wisdom of the Hakim

A sultan was on a ship with one of his best servants. The servant, who had never before taken a voyage—in fact, as a child of the mountains had never even seen the coast—sat in the empty belly of the ship and screamed, cried, trembled, and wailed. All were kind to him and tried to calm his fears, but their kindness reached only his ear, not his fearful heart. The ruler could hardly bear to hear the servant's cries any more, and the voyage through blue waters under blue sky was no longer a pleasure for him. Then the wise hakim, the physican, approached him and said, "Your Highness, with your permission, I can calm him down." Without a moment's hesitation, the sultan gave his permission. The hakim ordered the seamen to throw the servant overboard; the seamen did this to the crybaby only too gladly. The servant thrashed about in the water, grabbed for air, clutched the side of the ship, and begged that they take him on board again. So they pulled him up by his hair. From then on he sat very quietly in a corner. No one heard another word of fear come from his mouth. The sultan was amazed and asked the hakim, "What wisdom is contained in this action?"

The hakim answered, "He's never tasted the salt of the sea. And he didn't know how great the danger was in the water. So he couldn't know how wonderful it is to have the sturdy planks of the ship under him. Only he who has faced danger can know the value of peace and composure. You, who always have enough to eat, do not know the taste of country bread. The girl whom you do not consider pretty is my beloved. There is a difference

72

between a man who has his beloved beside him, and a man who expectantly longs for her arrival."

(After Saadi)

The knowledge of psychosomatic medicine—even if un-systematic—is not the only anticipation of modernism in ancient stories of the East. They show the beginnings of therapeutic processes that have first acquired form and scientific systematization in recent times. One sure process, used today mainly for treating anxieties, is behavior modification. It is based on the idea that behavior is learned and, accordingly, can be "unlearned" in a therapeutic situation.

This interchange of learning and unlearning accompanies our daily lives. To be sure, it can happen that we avoid situations that produce anxiety and thereby simply increase our anxieties. In behavior modification, the neurotic paradox is interrupted step by step, *e.g.*, by means of systematic desensitization. The goal is the realization that a situation or object need not always be accompanied by negative experiences. An example of ancient anxiety therapy is found in the story of the hakim's wisdom, as told by Saadi. In his time, concern with anxiety was not just a matter for the hakims, but was primarily a philosophical problem dealing with the essence of man. Anxiety was regarded as a reaction to man's relationship to the unknown. Eastern philosophers made distinctions among three kinds of anxieties, which they called primal anxieties. They are:

1) fear of the past, to which they attributed injustices and for which they required forgiveness and pardon as the treatment;

2) anxiety in the present, expressed by loneliness, which was to be eliminated by leaving the social arena and practicing asceticism;

3) fear of the future, expressed in feelings of meaninglessness and lack of goals. Prayer was recommened as an antidote.

In psychotherapy today, one again finds these three primal anxieties. Fear of the past and present are viewed as historically experienced anxieties. Fear of the future is placed in opposition to them as existential fear.

The systematization of anxiety and the teachings drawn from it can be understood against the religious cultural backgroud and are oriented more to that background than to actual observable character traits of man. Forgiveness is essentially a moral requirement of the highest sensitivity. As a rule, it assumes a certain degree of insight if it is not to lead merely to self-repudiation. This is why Hafis said, "If everyone knew everything about the other person, everyone would easily and gladly grant pardon."

Asceticism as an antidote for loneliness seems paradoxical, much like "committing suicide out of fear of dying." The idea behind it is that a person who voluntarily turns to asceticism, and sees in it a value that is also recognized by his environment and religion, can more easily take leave of his fear of loneliness. Asceticism can in the same way also mean escape, a reaction against fear of other people. Prayer and meditation as remedies for fear of the future have been recommended for centuries. They are considered agents of trust and hope. But this procedure becomes problematical if the demand for prayer prevents one from taking active measures for the future.

The "Healing" of the Caliph

A serious illness had struck the king. All attempts to cure him proved fruitless. The great and famous physician Rasi was finally called in for consultation. At first, he tried all the traditional methods of treatment, but without success. Finally Rasi asked the king to let him carry out the treatment as he thought best. The king, in his despair, gave his consent. Rasi asked the king to place two horses at his disposal. The fastest and the best Arabian horses were brought to him. Early the next day, Rasi ordered that the king be brought to the famous spa "Jouze Mullan," in Buchara. Since the king could not move, he was carried on a stretcher. At the spa, Rasi told the king to get undressed and ordered all the king's servants to get as far away from the spa as possible. The servants hesitated, but then drew back when the king let them know they should do as the hakim ordered.

Rasi had the horses tied at the entrance to the spa. Working with one of his pupils, he placed the king in a tub and quickly poured hot water over

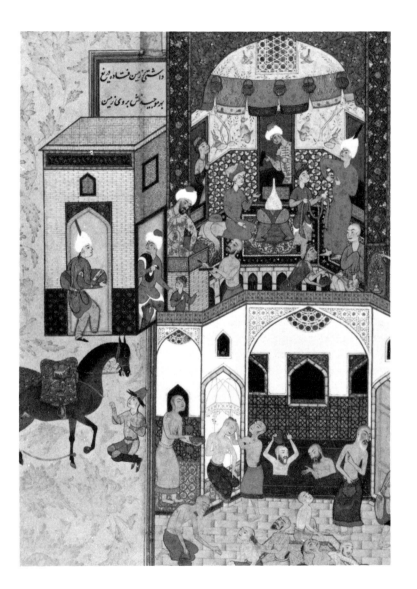

him. At the same time he fed him a hot syrup, which raised the sick man's temperature. After all this had happened, Rasi and his pupil got dressed. Rasi stood in front of the king and suddenly began to curse and insult him in the most horrible way. The king was shocked and became terribly upset over this rudeness and unjustified insult, especially because he was so helpless. In this state of upset, the king moved. When Rasi saw this, he drew out his knife, stepped close to the king, and threatened to kill him. Frightened, the king tried to save himself, until finally his fear suddenly gave him the strength to stand up and run away. At this moment, Rasi quickly left the room and, with his pupil, fled from the town on the horses.

The king collapsed in exhaustion. When he regained consciousness, he felt more free and was able to move. Still very angry, he called for his servant, got dressed, and rode back to his palace. The people gathered there rejoiced when they saw their king free of his ailment.

A week later, a letter from the physician reached the king. The letter contained these words of explanation: "I did everything I had learned as a doctor. When it produced no results, I artificially raised your temperature and by kindling your anger I gave you the strength to move your limbs. When I saw that your cure had begun, I left the city in order to escape your punishment. I ask you not to have me brought in, for I am aware of the unjust and vulgar insults I hurled at you in your helplessness and I am deeply ashamed of them." When the king heard this, deep gratitude filled his heart and he asked the doctor to come to him so that he could show his thanks.

Activating emotional participation is a very old procedure in medicine. So it was with Rhases (Rasi A.D. 850–923), the famous Persian physician, of whom it is said, among other things, that he was the first to use the word "psychotherapy."

His treatment was not "cathartic" in the actual sense of the word. The treatment did not take place by releasing an existent blockage of feeling. The congestion of feeling was first awakened by the insults and threats from Rasi, and introduced as the driving force in his cure. Rasi had taken care of the necessary prerequisites: The caliph had to be handed over to the hakim naked and helpless. Without these measures, the treatment would have surely become a double failure. The ruler would not have gotten himself into the excited condition that brought about his cure, for his servants would have prematurely and forcefully interrupted the therapeutic developments upon hearing his cries for help; Rasi would have had to fear for his own life.

As old as the story might be, it describes a problem of contemporary psychotherapy: Just like the caliph, our patients are surrounded by a crowd of allies, family members, friends, and their doctors who, in their mistrust, do not shy away from attempting to interrupt the treatment if the course of the treatment leads to crises or does not go according to their own views.

The Right Treatment

Karimkhan, the mighty ruler, was bedridden with illness, and all the doctors feared his rage. Finally, a servant used gentle force and great threats to bring a frightened hakim to the sickbed of the Karimkhan, who roared at him with a mighty voice and said, "You are known everywhere as a good doctor. Show your skill. But don't forget whom you have in front of you." The hakim carefully examined the doctor.

"Here, only one thing will help," he said. "Get everything ready for an enema."

"What? An enema?" screamed the king. "Who is supposed to have an enema?"

The frightful glance of the king made the hakim tremble. "The enema is for me, O lord." The king allowed it to take place, and look, from that hour on, the ruler's condition improved. And every time an illness plagued him, he summoned the hakim so that the doctor could have an enema.

From evening 'til morning he sat at the bed of the sick man and cried. The next morning he died, but the sick man kept on living.

(After Saadi)

A physician in the ancient East did not have it easy. His fee was usually a fee for success; mistakes in treatment were subject to revenge. Furthermore, the doctors faced the problem of everyone in the medical profession, namely, the responsibility for choosing among various risks. As servants of the great rulers, even the best doctors, like Avicena or Rasi, were subject to the whim of their masters. Along with worrying about the lives of their patients, they had to fear for their own lives.

Whoever Says *A* Must Also Say *B*

In a class known in the East as Maktab, the teacher had a lot of trouble with one boy. "Say **A***," {Persian:* **Alef***}. The boy just raised his head and shook it back and forth, clamping his lips together. The teacher exercised patience and started again, "You are such a nice boy—please say* **A**. *It won't hurt you." The only reply was an empty stare from the boy. Finally, after many attempts, the teacher lost his patience. "Say* **A***," he screamed, "say* **A**.*" But the boy's reply was only "Mm-mm." At that point, the teacher summoned the boy's father. Together they implored the little one to say* **A**. *Finally the boy gave in, and, to everyone's amazement, produced a clear and beautiful* **A**. *The teacher, surprised by this pedagogical success, cried, "Maschallah, how marvelous! Now say* **B***." But the boy protested violently and banged his little fists on the desk as he said, "Now that's enough. I knew what would happen to me if I just said* **A**. *Then you'd want me to say* **B***, and then I'd have to recite the whole alphabet, then learn to read and write and work arithmetic. I knew all along why I didn't want to say* **A***!"*

The boy knows what he wants. Since he can see the consequences of his action, he has an advantage over the adults. The ability to include the results of an action in one's considerations, even at the expense of spontaneity, proves not at all seldom to be very useful. What are the results for me, aside from pleasure, if I drink alcohol? What results must I count on if I cheat on my wife and take a mistress? What are the results if I eat too much? What are the results if I choose a political or religious concept?

Medicine, too, is faced with the task of saying *A* and accepting the corresponding consequences. We make choices like that when we adopt theoretical concepts. If we regard a certain illness to be inborn, there are different results from regarding it as acquired. If, for example, we include depression and schizophrenia among endogenous forms, the most appropriate therapy will be drug treatment. But if we assume that these illnesses are determined mainly by psychosocial causes, our first choice will by psychotherapy, environmental therapy, family therapy, and so forth.

While the relationship between diagnosis and forms of therapy is relatively straightforward in somatic medicine, basic decisions have to be made in psychosomatic medicine, psychiatry, and psychotherapy. These decisions have not yet been sufficiently proven scientifically and thus allow a wide margin for argument about belief and conviction.

The Shirt of a Happy Man

A caliph lay deathly ill on his silk cushions. The hakims, the physicians of his country, stood around him and agreed that only one thing could bring the caliph healing and salvation: placing under his head the shirt of a happy man. Messengers swarmed out looking in every city, every village, and every cottage for a happy man. But everyone they questioned had nothing but sorrow and worries. Finally, after giving up all hope, the messengers met a shepherd who laughed and sang as he watched his herds. Was he happy? "I can't imagine anyone happier than I," the shepherd replied, laughing.

"Then give us your shirt," cried the messengers. But the shepherd replied, "I don't have one." This pathetic news, that the only happy man the messengers had met did not own a shirt, gave the caliph cause for thought. For three days and three nights, he did not allow anyone to come to him. Finally, on the fourth day, he had his silk cushions and his precious stones distributed among the people, and, as the legend tells, from this time on the caliph was again healthy and happy.

(Eastern Story)

The doctors in this story want to use magic means, the shirt of a happy man. Ironically, it is not the shirt of the rich man, who would have to be able to afford to be happy. The story has the character of a didactic piece and is conspicuously ambiguous: On the one hand, the poor person who hears this story is depicted as the actual rich man who can finally afford to look down on the wealthy people. But, at the same time, the story has a smoothing quality: Don't get upset over social inequality; remember that you are blessed with other goods. Both interpretations show that a doctor's activities contain ideological elements alongside the healing ones. This does not mean that his activities are bad or objectionable. But it is important that he be aware of the philosophical, ideological assumptions so that he can avoid narrowmindedness.

Wealth frequently takes on a life of its own, be it as the prestige it transmits; the role behavior it demands; the exclusiveness it generates; or the quasi-Calvanistic ethic by which wealth must be taken care of and its development furthered like a child. In this way, a breach develops in the personality of a man, between his emotions, openness, and vulnerability on the one hand, and, on the other hand, the armor of his character, placed upon him by his social and economic position. Through this division, which strikes other people as artificial, some qualities, such as frugalness, achievement motivation, or even the need for contact, are sharply emphasized, at least insofar as it concerns people of the same class. But other qualities are brushed aside and seem to dwindle.

In the following Eastern story, in place of resignation and ironic protest, which contains a bit of necessity that can be turned into a virtue, we find the cunning of the mullah. He grabs the steer by the horns, joins the snob society a second time, despite all the insults, and opens their eyes.

The Hungry Caftan

Dressed in his modest and simple everyday robe, a mullah had gone to a party given by a highly respected citizen. All around him glittered the most beautiful clothes made of silk and velvet. The other guests looked disdainfully at his wretched clothes. They cut him dead, turned up their noses, and pushed him away from the magnificent foods on the buffet table. The mullah dashed home, put on his best caftan, and returned to the party, looking more noble than one of the caliphs. Oh, the fuss people made over him! Everyone tried to get into a conversation with him, or at least to snatch a word or two of his wise sayings. It was as if the cold buffet had been thought up just for him. From all sides, people offered him the tastiest dishes. But, instead of eating them, the mullah stuffed them into the wide sleeves of his caftan. Shocked as well as curious, the people stormed him with the question, "O lord, what are you doing there? Why don't you eat what we offer you?" The mullah kept stuffing his caftan and replied calmly, "I am an honest man, and, if we are honest, your hospitality isn't for me, but for my caftan. And it should have what it is entitled to."

3.

Sexuality and Marriage

The Sightseers and the Elephant

An elephant had been brought into a dark room at night for an exhibition. The people streamed by in throngs. Since it was dark, the visitors couldn't see the elephant; so, they tried to get an idea of his body by touching him. Because he was large, each visitor could only grab a part of the animal and describe it according to what he had felt. One of the visitors, who had gotten hold of a leg, explained that the elephant was like a mighty pillar; a second one, who touched a tusk, described the elephant as a pointy object; a third, who grabbed the creature's ear, claimed he was not different from a fan; the fourth, who ran his hand over the elephant's back, stated that the elephant was as flat as a couch.

(After Mowlana)

A fifty-year-old worker had come to me for treatment because of marital problems and professional difficulties. Already at the first session, he got around to talking about a problem that obviously bothered him. "I become very sexually aroused at the sight of a woman or girl in a raincoat made of rubber, patent leather, or plastic. Only when my wife wears shiny black sex clothes am I able to accept her as a woman. My wife used to go along with all that, and I ordered all the rubber and patent leather articles from

82

England. But for a while now she's been reluctant to wear those things. Since then our marriage just hasn't been right."

In handling this case, it would have been logical to focus the treatment on the fetishism that is hidden behind these wishes, and to relate all questions and possible solutions to the problem "rubber clothing." But, in the spirit of "positive psychotherapy," I proceeded differently. It struck me that in the patient's relationship with his wife, nothing seemed to move him except her willingness to adapt to his sexual wishes. For this reason, I was especially interested in the concepts that had formed the basis of his upbringing. There were clearly a number of clues which could be useful in explaining and understanding his problem.

"At home, the main thing was that we always be clean and adroit. My mother always said, 'Man is received according to his clothing and let go according to his spirit.' That made a big impression on me. Today it is still hard for me to accept people who don't wear ties, who are unshaved, or who are otherwise not dressed properly." He had carried this wish for "correct clothing" even into sexuality and was so bound by this idea that basically he felt attracted only by the external qualities of rubber clothing, but not by the body and personality of his wife. Since I had noticed how open he was to fantasy, I had already told him the story of "The Sightseers and the Elephant" at our first session.

The patient mulled over this story for a long time. Frequently he told me he had been thinking about it. But a few weeks passed before he told me the results of his considerations: "By my wanting to see my wife in shiny black sex clothes, the desire to see her only in that way was so strongly defined that her personality faded more and more into the background. Her eyes and face I actually didn't see anymore. To a certain extent, she had just become a clothes hanger for the sex clothing. The totality of her presence was lost, just as the sightseers saw only a certain part of the elephant and saw him the way they had expected to."

In a certain way the patient mapped out the strategy for his own treatment, the main features of which were the extension of his goals: In dealing with business partners, he wanted to see the total conduct of the people, not just their adherence to formal rules of courtesy, not just whether they wore a tie; he did not want to just see sex clothing, but to accept his wife as she was. The patient then tried on his own to experience his wife, his surroundings, business partners, and colleagues in a new way. For him this was a voyage of discovery into a previously almost unknown land. Repeatedly he came to our sessions and told of new discoveries: that it had been good for him, and had yielded no disadvantages, to express his opinions to his boss; that he had had lively and stimulating conversations with colleagues whom he'd previously dealt with only on a business level; what physical qualities he had been able to find in his wife, what features he admired in her, and what common interests they had recently developed.

In the sense of positive processes, the fetishism and the fixation with hedonistic, supple, rubber clothes had receded into the background. Thus the way was opened up for treating his problem, whereby fetishism was only the tip of the iceberg of an even more comprehensive conflict situation.

A Story on the Way

Persian mysticism tells of a wanderer who trudged along on a seemingly endlessly long road. He was loaded down with all sorts of burdens. A heavy sack of sand hung on his back; a thick water hose was draped around his body. In his right hand, he carried an oddly shaped stone, in the left hand a boulder. Around his neck an old millstone dangled on a frayed rope. Rusty chains, with which he dragged heavy weights through the dusty sand, wound around his ankles. On his head, the man was balancing a half-rotten pumpkin. With every step he took, the chains rattled. Moaning and groaning, he moved forward step by step, complaining of his hard fate and the weariness that tormented him. On his way, a farmer met him in the glowing heat of midday. The farmer asked, "Oh, tired wanderer, why do you load yourself down with this boulder?"

"Awfully dumb," replied the wanderer, "but I hadn't noticed it before." With that, he threw the rock away and felt much lighter.

Again, after going a long way down the road, a farmer met him and asked, "Tell me, tired wanderer, why do you trouble yourself with the half-

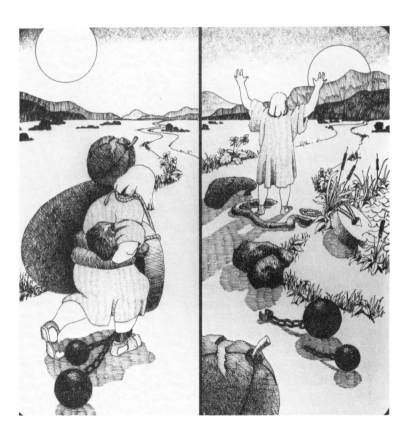

rotten pumpkin on your head, and why do you drag those heavy iron weights behind you on chains?"

The wanderer answered, "I'm very glad you pointed it out to me. I didn't realize what I was doing to myself." He took off the chains and smashed the pumpkin into the ditch alongside the road. Again, he felt lighter. But the farther he went, the more he began to suffer again.

A farmer coming from the field watched him in amazement and said, "Oh, good man, you are carrying sand in the sack, but what you see far off in the distance is more sand than you could ever carry. And your big water hose—as if you planned to cross the Kawir Desert. All the while there's a clear stream flowing alongside you, which will accompany you on your way for a long time." Upon hearing this, the wanderer tore open the water hose and emptied its brackish water onto the path. Then he filled a hole with the sand from his knapsack. He stood there pensively and looked into the sinking sun. The last rays sent their light to him. He glanced down at himself, saw the heavy millstone around his neck and suddenly realized it was the stone that was still causing him to walk so bent over. He unloosened it and threw it as far as he could into the river. Freed from his burdens, he wandered on through the cool of the evening to find lodging.

In the course of his treatment, a fifty-one-year-old depressed patient set about to read my book *Psychotherapy of Everyday Life*. As often happens, he started at the end of the book and read the "Story on the Way." At the next session, the patient was very animated. He bubbled over with a number of experiences and habits that he considered burdens: "A word of advice in my upbringing was 'Be frugal!' And that advice still haunts me today. In trying to be frugal, I make such a mess of things that this form of frugality is, in the end, too expensive. Here's an example: I go into the cellar to get something from my workshop, but, to save money, I turn on only the stairs light and hunt around in the half-dark workshop, but don't find what I'm looking for. Then I turn on the light and find it immediately. My excessive frugality has cost me unnecessary time and frustration. Even the principle 'Be careful and think of safety' is occasionally a burden for me. Although I am skilled with my hands, I don't dare rebuild a cabinet, because I'm afraid something could go wrong. I keep putting off doing it, and this, too, makes me feel burdened. After a while, I go ahead and start the work, and I succeed in doing it. Afterwards I have the feeling that my excessive need for security and my fear of doing something wrong or messing something up are almost like the half-rotten pumpkin on the wanderer's head. But, all by myself, I've been able to come to terms with some of these stresses, and I'm very proud of that. My parents were very upset about the construction of our house, since I could hardly handle the financial burden. Again and again, they said to me, 'Take the safe way.' But I had courage, and my labor and my wife's help made it possible to reach our goal. The house is finished now, and the debts are all paid off except for a few mortgage payments. But, even so, I still carry burdens like stones and chains around my neck, burdens I've in part recognized and would like to throw off, like the wanderer on his way."

About the Fortune of Having Two Wives

A sheik had the greatest luck on earth: He had two wives. Feeling excessively happy, he went to the bazaar and bought two identical gold necklaces, which he presented to his wives after some happy hours with them. The only stipulation was that each wife had to promise not to tell the other one. But not every earthly joy remains untroubled. One day the wives, excited by rivalry and jealousy, came to him and bombarded him with questions. "Tell us, most splendid of all men, whom do you like of us the best?"

"My darlings, I love the two of you more than anything," the sheik defended himself appeasingly.

"No, no," protested the women, "We want to know from you which one of us receives your greater love."

"But my pets, why do you want dissatisfaction? I have both of you in my heart." But the women weren't satisfied with that.

"You won't get away from us. Come on; speak up. Who is the queen of your heart?"

Since he could no longer submit to the oppressive questions of his wives, he lowered his voice promisingly and whispered, "If you absolutely have to know, I will tell you the truth. The one I love the most is the one I gave the

87

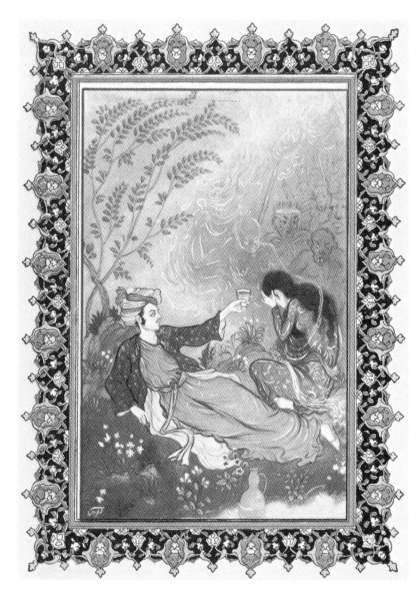

golden chain to." Both women looked at each other victoriously and were satisfied.

(Persian Story)

Completely unraveled, crying, and trembling all over, a forty-one-year-old academician came to my office. At the start of our conversation, he said repeatedly, "I can't go on living. I want to die." Then he explained: "I'm suffering from sudden occurring attacks of anxiety and restlessness, accompanied by an immediate drop in blood pressure. This leads to a great sense of insecurity, since these conditions come on at any time and without warning. My physical capabilities have declined. Feelings of restlessness occur particularly strongly and spontaneously in the car, when I have to wait at a red light. I find waiting very difficult. I avoid waiting rooms of any kind as much as I can."

There then occurred a functionally induced heart irregularity. The clinical examination that followed immediately revealed no basis for organic damage. The irregularity began at two o'clock in the afternoon and stopped spontaneously at 10:00 P.M., while the patient was still in the clinic. The patient was released from the clinic after a week's stay, but his condition became visibly worse.

"I prefer to be alone. I become terribly upset by sudden occurrences (doorbells, unannounced visitors, bad news, and so on). With increasing frequency, I have to trade my office for my bed. (I'm self-employed.) I start brooding, and suddenly I'm thinking about the meaning of life. I can't live any longer. I want to die."

For a long time, I could get nothing from him except these stereotyped statements. But, gradually, he began to talk about being in a conflict and not seeing a way out of it. His conflict can be summarized as follows: Married, the father of two children, professionally quite successful, he had met another woman and now had to decide between her and his wife. He found himself now, to his misfortune, in the happy circumstance of having gotten along well with his wife and children for a long time. This fact meant that he did not have an excuse, which would have made it easier for him to leave his family.

His wife, who placed great importance on fidelity and did not

89

want an unfaithful marriage, had found out about the affair and demanded he make a choice. For many reasons, his conflict was particularly painful for him. He considered the consequences of a separation for his family, himself, his wife, children, relatives, his career, and his future. At the same time, he also thought about how much he cared for his girlfriend and did not want to hurt her, because this would have pained him, too. This problem, with all its pros and cons, occupied him day and night. Even when he himself did not think about it, his wife approached him about it, or he was reminded of it by his girlfriend. All arguments had lost their logical sequence and whirled around in his brain. His whole life was focused on the decision that he could not make. Despite his desire for help, he was moved by deep pessimism: "I've thought about it for weeks and months," he said. "I've looked for solutions that seemed reasonable to me, but that has not helped. My friends, to the extent that they know about it, have given me advice. But my emotions don't stop with the suggestions. They are as mixed up as I am."

The patient was in a severe depression and dangerously suicidal. Not to give him advice or show him a solution, but in order to lead him away from his intensive and endless brooding, I told him the story "About the Fortune of Having Two Wives."

The patient began to smile, shook his head lightly, and said, "I used to also think it would be fortunate to have two wives. Before falling asleep, I've imagined what it would be like to be spoiled by two women." At this session and in the following ones, we talked about why he had this desire, what criteria he had used in selecting his wife, and what characteristics his girlfriend had. We discussed the fact that, when there were fights with his wife, he imagined things would be better with a different woman, and that he had nourished this idea in fantasies and daydreams. We also talked about why he was finding it so hard to decide whether to leave his wife or give up his girlfriend.

In these conversations we also dealt with the deeper psychodynamic backgrounds and contents involved. These talks helped him bring some sense of order to his experience and to make an independent decision based on them. As he informed me, he finally decided in favor of his wife and family, chiefly because he saw no possibility for "peaceful coexistence."

But this concrete decision was not the goal of the treatment. In coming to this decision, in fact, the patient had turned away from the actual conflict and the particular meaning of fidelity. Other areas of conflict dealing with issues peculiar to personality had been taken up. Against the background of these conflicts, the psychosomatics had developed.

In psychotherapeutic practice, mating and marriage are sometimes reflected in a completely differently manner from what morality and good manners would dictate. It seems as if marriage, faithfulness, and partnership are not what they claim to be. This difference between what is and what should be becomes apparent when one knows the background and conditions that lead to catastrophic problems in relationships. These conditions are not just in the person's internal world, in the unconscious and uncontrolled past, and also not just in the external reality, in social, economic, and communal relationships, but rather in the close connection between the inner and outer.

Nietzsche describes the desolate situation of a marriage from the woman's view. He writes, "And it's even better to break a marriage than to bend it, or to live a lie. Thus spoke a woman: I probably broke the marriage, but first the marriage broke me."

The Dirty Nests

A dove was constantly changing her nest. The strong smell that the nests had developed over time was unbearable for her. She complained about this bitterly as she spoke with a wise, old, and experienced dove. The latter nodded his head several times and said, "By changing your nest all the time, you don't change anything. The smell that bothers you does not come from the nests, but from you."

A well-known, successful journalist came to me at the advice of an acquaintance, a doctor who had dealt with psychotherapeutic problems in his work. The journalist had a very sporty appearance,

91

was slender and sinewy, and showed a self-confidence that one rarely finds in patients. He quickly got to the point: He had been married six times. His current wife had also been divorced several times. But now a problem had emerged for which he sought professional help. His wife was terribly jealous and never let him go off by himself. For this reason, he felt very confined. This conduct on the part of his wife hampered both his private and professional life. It was not hard for him to concede that his wife's jealousy was not just a fantasy of hers. He had given her good cause to be jealous. He ended by saying, "I want to be free again and feel that I'm free."

We talked about his previous marriages and divorces. His current wife had left her husband because of him, just as he had gotten a divorce for her. The reason was that he had felt tied down by his wife and was attracted by the relatively open-minded attitudes of the woman who became his sixth wife. For the journalist, the situation was clear: The problem was with his wives; again and again he had been forced to realize that he had not yet found the right woman. It seemed to me that he had sought therapeutic help because, unconsciously, he was looking for an ally, someone who would stand by and support him with psychological tricks as he tried to leave his wife. But on the other hand, the patient's recurring problem could not be ignored. For this reason I confronted him with the story of the dirty nests. The journalist seemed surprised. He was silent for a while, which indicated that the story was working in him. It looked as if I had pulled the rug out from under him; at the same time, it seemed that I had touched on something that bothered him, something he had not dared to face himself. Finally he said, "I can imagine why you told me the story. I am the stinking bird, and the nests are my wives. Wherever I settle down in marriage, it soon reeks from trouble. I always thought my wives were at fault. Now I'd like to know why I should be responsible for this smell?" This question was the theme of our further discussions. The patient told of an inner battle concerning his parents. His father had owned a circus and had traveled from place to place. Since his mother never took part in these tours, the patient had frequently come to a "substitute mother," his father's girlfriends. This atmosphere of free-wheeling change of location and partner seemed to him to be the epitome of an independent and free life. He explained, "Journalism as a profession comes closest to life in the circus. Here, I have my freedom and can devote myself to my main interests, namely foreign peoples, their customs and problems."

We talked about the fact that he acted this way in order to be loved, but that for his part he was afraid of and avoided intimate situations that he had to endure passively. This particular therapy session was a single intervention treatment, for the patient's foreign assignments made it impossible for him to have psychotherapy on a regular basis. Prospects for concrete results in this short treatment were relatively slim. Nevertheless, our conversation, particularly the story of the dirty nests, continued to have an effect on the patient. Weeks later, he called me and explained that he found himself thinking a lot about our session and the story. The problem of his relationships had acquired new aspects.

The journalist's tendency to attribute problems to deficiencies in his female partners and to deny his own responsibility in the conflict is a psychological resistance, which we encounter in many forms. It is a matter of projections of conflict contents, which are not seen in the person himself, but in others. This leads to generalization of conflicts, with the goal of protecting one's own ego.

One tries to escape his conflicts, but he carries them around nevertheless, like a donkey with his burden, and finds them at every place and with every new partner. On this subject, Wilhelm Busch once said, "The place is good, the time is new. The old rascal is there again." Under these conditions, self-help is sometimes impossible, namely when one confuses the essential with the nonessential and is happy to deal with conflicts that, compared to the real problem, are only minor. Saadi expressed this in the following verses: "The sheik is constantly busy with worrying about the decor and rearrangement of his palace. In doing so, he overlooks the fact that from the foundation upward, his palace is not in good shape and that there are cracks in the walls."

Two Friends and Four Women

"How wonderful it is to have two women," a man raved to one of his friends as the two smoked a waterpipe in a coffeehouse. With the most flowery words he praised the variety and the magnificence of experiencing the fact that two blossoms can smell so different. The friend's eyes became bigger and bigger. My friend must have it as good as in paradise, *he thought to himself.* Why shouldn't I also taste the honey of two women as my friend here probably does? *Soon after that, he married a second woman. When he tried to share the bed with her on their wedding night, she rejected him angrily. "Let me sleep," she said, "Go to your first wife. I don't want to be a fifth wheel. Either me or your other wife." To find consolation, he went to his other wife. But when he tried to slip into bed next to her, she complained, "Not with me. If you have married a second woman and I'm not enough for you, just go back to her." There was nothing left for him to do but leave his own house and go to the nearby mosque to find a place to sleep there. When he tried to fall asleep in a praying position, he heard someone clearing his throat behind him. Astonished, he turned around, for the person who had just arrived was none other than his good friend who had raved about how wonderful it was to have two wives. "Why did you come here?" he asked him, amazed.*

"My wives wouldn't let me get near them. That's been going on for several weeks."

"But why did you tell me how great it is to live with two women?" Ashamed, the friend answered, "I felt so lonesome in this mosque and wanted to have a friend with me."

For good reason, psychoanalysis recommends that the therapist's private life and his therapeutic work with the patients be kept separate. Almost all patients show a childlike need to learn about the therapist's private life and to identify with him. This tendency leads to special problems, which are sometimes not easy to solve.

After changing residences, a thirty-two-year-old economist came to me for group therapy. Prior to this, he had been in individual therapy for some time. In the course of the group's work, a female patient began talking about how hurt she was by her husband's infidelity. While some members of the group, mainly

94

married women, proclaimed their solidarity, the economist took a counter-position in saying, "I'm married, too, and for a long time I've been wanting to have a girlfriend. I imagine it would really be fantastic to have such a real diversion from the dreariness of everyday married life." (The group became restless; most of the men present and some of the women began to laugh, others to protest vehemently, and the patient who brought up the issue in the first place was silent.) The following dialog develops between members of the group and the man.

MEMBER: What led you to feel this way? Do you have so many problems with your wife?

MAN: Actually, things are okay. Of course, we always have ordinary things we fight about, but otherwise we get along pretty well. But what bothers me the most is that my wife is almost pathologically jealous.

FEMALE MEMBER: I don't think it is at all right that you want to cheat on your wife.

MAN: Why not? My last therapist also had a girlfriend, and that made a big impression on me.

There then developed a debate on the pros and cons of promiscuity. When the group became lively, I told them the story of the good fortune of having two wives. I told them the story instead of giving an outright interpretation of what was going on.

The story accomplished two things within the group. The participants calmed down, and the way was paved for discussion about imitation and identification and the concept of fidelity.

Marriage as a Flower

Frequently, married people tired of the marriage seek therapeutic help. Monotony has crept into their everyday lives, and this monotony causes almost everything, even tenderness, sexuality, and intimate conversation, to become routine. Quite often both partners react to such a situation with desperation, depression, and resignation. From the fact that the relationship

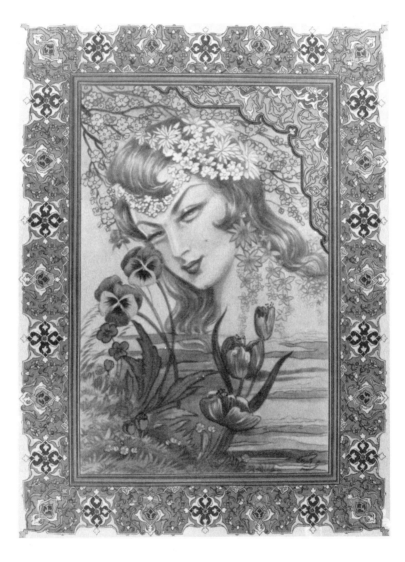

is problematical, it is concluded that the two don't really suit each other. There's nothing to say to the other person; regardless of how badly one wants a point of contact, he seems to encounter nothing but inner desolation and emptiness.

In such a situation, the following dialog took place with forty-three-year-old female patient. She had complained of the lack of dialog and the monotony in her marriage, as well as her own shortcomings with respect to creativity and responsiveness. I asked the patient what she would do if she had a beautiful potted plant, such as a fuchsia.

Therapist: How do you take care of this plant?

The patient shook her head in amazement as if she could not understand what this question had to do with her marriage. "If I had such a flower, I would water it at regular intervals." The patient loved flowers and gave the question some more thought. "After six months or a year I'd change the flowerpot and give the plant new soil. In between, I might add fertilizer again. And then I'd put it on the windowsill, where it would get enough light."

At this point I interrupted the patient and asked her, "And what do you do with your marriage?"

This question visibly startled the woman. I noticed that she realized the discrepancy between the intensive, loving care she'd give to the flowers and the loveless way she treated her marriage. With this in mind, she said, "If my marriage were a flower, it would have withered and died a long time ago." The patient began to transfer the image of the flower to her marriage. She remarked, "If we did just a little more for each other every day, perhaps exchanging compliments or at least acknowledging each other's achievements, that would be water for our marriage." For a long time she just sat there and thought. "Actually I've neglected myself a lot, too. I must admit, a new dress, a different hairdo, or makeup have not interested me for a while. To be very blunt, I simply didn't have the desire to make myself beautiful for my husband. The same is probably true for him. Something like that would be the fertilizer for my marriage."

At subsequent sessions, the patient again and again returned to the image of the flower. She told of how she and her husband had, to some extent, isolated themselves in their house. She thought that perhaps a vacation could be a "change of flowerpot" for them. Guests and friends could form the soil in the flowerpot and dispel their isolation and their problems in establishing social contact.

Conversations such as these showed that progress had been made in that the patient no longer experienced her marriage as vaguely unsatisfying; by using the metaphor of the flowerpot, she was able to concretize her general feelings through examples and descriptions. Viewed in this way, her situation was no longer so helpless. The couple now had a better grasp of their situation and could work toward saving their relationship.

Comparisons Limp

There once came to a doctor a cobbler who suffered from severe pains and seemed to be dying. The doctor checked him carefully, but could not find a prescription that would have helped him. The patient asked anxiously, "Is there nothing else that can save me?"

The physician answered the cobbler by saying, "Unfortunately, I know of no other means."

Upon hearing that, the cobbler replied, "If there is nothing left, I have just one final wish. I'd like a cooking pot with two kilos of thick beans and a liter of vinegar."

The doctor shrugged his shoulders with resignation and said, "I don't think much of that idea, but, if you think it will work, go ahead and try." Throughout the night the doctor waited for news of the man's death. But the next morning, to the doctor's amazement, the cobbler was alive and kicking. The doctor wrote in his journal, "Today a cobbler came to me for whom nothing could be done. But two kilos of beans and a liter of vinegar have helped him."

Shortly afterwards, the doctor was called to help a deathly ill tailor. In this case, the doctor was again at his wit's end. As an honest man, he admitted this to the tailor. The ailing man begged, "But don't you know of any other possible cure?"

The doctor thought a minute and said, "No, but recently a cobbler came to me with similar complaints. He was helped by two kilos of beans and a liter of vinegar."

"Well, if there's no other remedy, I'll just try that one," replied the tailor. He ate the beans with vinegar and was dead by the next day. At that point, the doctor wrote in his journal, "Yesterday a tailor came to me. Nothing could be done for him. He ate two kilos of beans with a liter of vinegar and then he died. What's good for cobblers is not good for tailors."

Each of us discovers for himself that some things are easier than others, that he is more interested in some things than in others, and that he has his own individual talents. Although many things in our society—even the way we perceive ourselves and others—are defined by comparisons, we are not all the same. While people all have much in common, there are also considerable differences.

A thirty-two-year-old female journalist once complained, in a therapy group for women, "Something's wrong with my sexuality. I'm not normal. I think I'm frigid. . . ."

The other members of the group listened with interest. One of them, Mrs. T., asked spontaneously, "What makes you think so?"

The patient: "I've always had that feeling. But I noticed it in particular after I had a conversation with my girl friend. We had been talking about an article on orgasm that had just appeared in a magazine. She began telling me how she was in seventh heaven every time she had sex, that she had to shout for pure joy, and that an orgasm was the greatest experience for her. She could sometimes hardly wait to get home. She says that sometimes she has sex three or four times a day. Compared to her, I don't seem to have much feeling."

Mrs. T: "What's an orgasm like for you?"

Patient: "I've only been in bed with my husband. We have sex about twice a week. It's not unpleasant for me. To be perfectly honest, it's even fun, but somehow I've never had that great experience. I do have feelings similar to an orgasm, sometimes even several times during sex, but I don't believe it can compare with the genuine orgasms my girl friend has."

As a therapist, I did not try to explain the patient's comments. Instead I told the entire group the story "Comparisons Limp." Afterwards the scene became very lively. One patient said she didn't enjoy sex at all. A forty-nine-year-old woman claimed, "At my age, sex isn't a problem anymore. For me, it is more important to live in peace with my husband and to have the feeling that we are there for each other."

Suddenly it was clear to the group that each person has his own way of experiencing things, and that everyone is stamped by his own problems, discoveries and questions. The group discussion revolved around the theme "Uniqueness." Experiences and fantasies related to this theme were shared by everyone.

Iron Is Not Always Hard

In connection with the selective sexual disorder that often disturbs the sexual relationship with certain partners—usually the spouse—I almost regularly hear the complaint, "We are completely different people; we aren't right for each other." This idea has a lot to do with marital problems. It runs counter to the concept of expansion: "Sameness brings us into a state of quiet. Contradiction is what makes us productive." (Goethe)

While the comment "We don't suit each other" already points to the dissolution of the relationship, the principle of expansion tries to achieve a delay. People try to open up their hardened defenses and to question the prejudices and mutual assessments that have existed for years.

Counter to this openness, there is the protest "The problems have existed for years, and I don't see why they should disappear now; my partner will never change."

While treating a patient who had expressed similar thoughts, I described the following image. It made her very pensive and caused her to reassess her relationship with her partner. *"Look at this piece of iron,"* I said as I showed her a cast iron sculpture on my desk. *"This iron is gray, tough, cold, and sharp-edged. When it is heated, it loses these characteristics. It is no longer gray, tough, cold, and sharp-edged, but*

100

glowing white, fluid, hot, and without a definite form. To a certain extent it has taken on the qualities of the fire."

For the patient, this meant that her husband's "sharp-edged" manner was not an unchangeable personal trait, but depended on the situation and on the patient herself. Because of his profession, he had less time for his wife than she wanted. She reacted to this with complaints and open refusals. As a result, the man sought other partners from time to time, aggravated his wife with his excessive frugality, and more and more frequently avoided her. To put it into images: The iron had grown cold. In order to forge it again, it had to be reheated. This was a task which the woman had to take up within her therapy.

Fifty Years of Politeness

An elderly couple celebrated their golden anniversary after long years of marriage. While eating breakfast together, the woman thought, "For fifty years I've always been considerate of my husband and have always given him the crusty top of the breakfast roll. Today I want finally to enjoy this delicacy for myself." She spread the top part with butter and gave the other part to her husband. Contrary to her expectations, he was very pleased, kissed her hand, and said, "My darling, you've just given me the greatest joy of the day. For over fifty years I haven't eaten the bottom part of the roll, which is the part I like best. I always thought you should have it because you like it so much."

Instead of setting goals for ourselves, we sometimes take on goals that are set for us by others: "I always go according to what my husband wants." We let ourselves be led by what we think are the wishes and intentions of our partner. We thereby renounce our own initiative and neglect our own needs—obviously without reason. This politeness, the silencing of our own needs and wishes, leads not only to misunderstandings, but also to narrow divisions of roles, which, in the course of time, can seem like burdens and a lack of freedom.

Here is a report from a forty-five-year-old housewife, the mother of two children, who was treated for depression, anxiety, stomach and intestinal troubles, and circulatory problems.

"I always used to be considerate of other people—my husband, children, parents, relatives, acquaintances, neighbors, and so forth. I wanted to do things right for everyone. But I just ended up with a totally disturbed relationship with myself. On top of this, there was my problem in making a decision. I always reached a decision by saying, 'What will the others say?' 'Is it okay with them?' 'What do they think?' 'Are they satisfied?' But if I made a decision and saw that someone didn't agree with it, I withdrew it immediately and did things I didn't want to do at all. I was constantly plagued with doubts and feelings of guilt. Disagreements around me disturbed me a lot. I was terribly dependent on the opinions and good wishes of others. Furthermore, I had taken on so much work that I simply couldn't deal with. The housework grew to be an insurmountable obstacle. I gave up, lost all courage, and succumbed to anxiety and depression, which were treated with medication. If I was at the end of my rope, I went to bed. When I had recovered physically and emotionally, it all started over again. If my condition got worse, I took medicine for anxiety and depression. I slowly began to feel that I was perhaps melancholic and couldn't get along without these drugs. Whenever things didn't go right, when I didn't do something to my husband's satisfaction, when he reprimanded me, I just gave in rather than talk about it. I always said, 'Why bother? There's no point to it.' I lost more and more self-confidence, had no initiative any more; it was all the same to me.

"Whenever I was again at the end of my rope, I didn't try to spare myself, but just kept going until I couldn't do any more. It was like a compulsion. A voice inside me said, 'You have to,' and another voice said, 'I can't. I don't want to anymore.' Ferocious battles took place in me. I was so preoccupied with myself and my complaints and problems that I often couldn't think about anything else.

"In therapy the scales fell from my eyes. I suddenly realized I can be free, too, and that it is just up to me to achieve it. Only now do I fully realize what pressure I lived under all those years."

102

A fifty-two-year-old woman experienced great anxieties when she had to separate from her adult son. She complained that she had lost the ground under her feet. "Sometimes I'm overcome by the feeling that I've lived in vain. This happens when I think about my current situation. What have I accomplished in my life, and what do I really mean to my son? He hardly ever shows his face around here." At this point the concept of the woman clearly emerged: "Since I don't have my son (children) around here any more, my life is meaningless. I am worthless."

To counter this idea, I told the patient a parable:

The Secret of the Seed

A seed offers itself for the tree which grows from it. Seen externally, the seed is lost, but the same seed that is sacrificed is embodied in the tree, its branches, blossoms, and fruits. If the continued existence of that seed had not been sacrificed for the tree, no branches, blossoms, or fruits could have developed.

(After 'Abdu'l-Bahá)

The patient accepted this mythology as flattery, as an honor bestowed on her for her conduct. She was the one who had sacrificed herself and renounced her own interests, but had finally achieved her son's being able to lead an independent and happy life. It did the patient good that her achievement was recognized. Only after her personal accomplishment was confirmed and she could feel secure in this recognition, was she finally in a position to give up, step by step, her fixation with her singular and dominant reason for living, namely her son. This dissolution was no longer just a negative process for her, a contradiction of the maternal role. It was a step on the way to new interests and new goals.

The Sparrow-Peacock

A sparrow wanted to be like a peacock. How impressed he was by the proud gait of the great bird, the high-held head, the mighty wheel he made with his tail! "I want to be like that, too," said the sparrow. "The admiration of all the others will surely be mine." He stretched his head upward, breathed in deeply so that his tiny breast expanded, spread out his tailfeathers and tried to run as elegantly as he had seen the peacock do. He stumbled back and forth and felt terribly proud. But, after he had done this awhile, he found that the unusual posture was a real exertion. His neck hurt, his feet hurt, and the worst was that the other birds, the puffed-up blackbirds, the canaries in all their finery, and the stupid ducks, all laughed at the sparrow-peacock. Soon it became too much for him.

I don't like this game anymore, he thought to himself. I'm tired of being a peacock. I want to act like a sparrow again. But, when he tried to run like a sparrow again, he couldn't. Instead of running as he used to, he suddenly hopped around and could do nothing else. This is how sparrows learned to hop.

A forty-year-old Persian woman, the wife of a businessman, had come to me during a trip to Europe. She was suffering from depression, sleep disorders, and intestinal problems for which she had already been examined and treated in Iran and in the United States. She said, "I wake up early, but stay in bed 'till around ten o'clock. I feel very lonely. I always ask myself why I should get up early. After all, my children aren't there. I no longer accept invitations. I prefer to stay home. I start crying for no reason and can't stop. I don't take baths anymore, don't comb my hair, and could care less about clothes, although that was all different before. I'm very nervous. When the phone rings, I almost have a heart attack. I immediately jump up and think, *That's my son in America.* My husband is very kind to me. But I don't know why I have less and less to do with him." The patient, the mother of three children, had suffered from these symptoms since her youngest son, at her urging, had been sent to the United States to study, when he was sixteen years old. During our conversation, she kept coming back to her older sister, who, from all appearances, was her most important role model and her greatest rival. The sister had married a diplomat and could thus visit various countries, including the United States. For the patient, travel became the epitome of the ideal lifestyle, one that she would gladly have adopted. But, because of her husband, she was tied to Iran. In her place, two of her sons traveled abroad. The oldest studied in Germany, and the youngest studied in the United States and lived with her sister in Beverly Hills. Of this youngest son, the mother had said, "He's much different from my other sons. Through his manner, he makes being at home very pleasant." With two sons abroad, the patient had a good excuse to travel. She visited her son in the United States for three months and her son in Germany for two. During this time, the latter became her chauffeur, driving her from one doctor to another, using up his vacation time and even having to take a month off without pay.

Because of her visit, there were conflicts between the son and his German wife, who could not understand this form of maternal love. Despite the fulfillment of all her wishes, the patient felt anything but happy. Neither America nor Europe had lived up to her expectations. Her conflict of wanting to be like her sister had not been resolved in the way she had hoped.

Despite her exact depiction of her situation, the patient kept attributing her illness to organic causes. Since I was more and more convinced that the conflict with her sister played a key role, I told her the story of the sparrow-peacock.

The patient seemed unpleasantly moved, but immediately diverted the conversation to the problems her son was having in college, and tried to avoid the ideas contained in the story.

At the beginning of the next session she asked me, "What did you mean to say with that story?"

I replied, "How did you understand the story?"

She: "I don't like the story. I don't think it is flattering to me. I see myself as the sparrow-peacock, as the sparrow that wants to imitate the peacock and in the end can only hop around. . . . The peacock is my sister, I'm the sparrow. . . . I have always admired and imitated my sister."

A few minutes later she said, "I have a very kind and dear husband. Financially we are very well off. We aren't as rich as my sister, but we can afford a lot of things. To be perfectly honest, after being in the United States, I'm not sure my sister is really content."

The patient gained more and more insight into the fact that she had expended a great deal of herself in trying to be like her sister and to achieve what she had done. Since her treatment, as emergency treatment, could last for only three sessions, only this level of the therapy could be worked out more intensively. For purposes of self-help, which was to take over the function of further therapy, we were concerned with expanding the goal. What goals and wishes did the woman have besides the futile wish to be like her sister? Most of all, she wanted societal interests—the education of children and the advancement of socially disadvantaged children. We systematically discussed the various possibilities that existed. In our correspondence, which continues to this day, I hear from time to time of her activities and successes in newly opened areas. She has even been able to stimulate her husband's interest in them.

4.

Stories in Psychotherapy

Courage for Truth

When Mohammed was in flight and everyone was looking for him, Ali, his son-in-law, had an idea of how to save him. He hid the prophet in a tall basket, put the heavy load on his head, and balanced it as he walked out between the guards at the city gate. "What do you have in the basket?" asked a customs guard sternly. "Mohammed the Prophet," Ali replied to him. The guards, who mistook this truth for a quick-witted display of cheekiness, laughed and allowed Ali and the prophet in the basket to pass by.

Ali's trick—defending himself with the truth because of its unbelievability and improbability—is still used where the truth can produce unpleasant results. This is also true for psychiatry and psychotherapy, which, despite all enlightenment, are still tainted with the image of the insane asylums of bygone times. Even if the analyst, in many circles, is part of the good life, included as a status symbol under the title "my analyst," the general opinion about psychiatry and psychotherapy is still quite behind the times. As a result, many patients try to keep their visits to the therapist a deep secret. Outwardly they reveal nothing because they are afraid of being considered abnormal, sick, or conflict-laden. They fear it may be damaging to their careers. This problem is particularly acute for the members of the middle class.

A highly regarded judge once invited me to a festive party. He had come to me for help much earlier because of problems with his son. In many respects the situation at the party was rather tense. The other guests were all attorneys, judges, and lawyers. I was the only therapist. The host, my former patient, seemed to carry this tension around with him. When he was taking my coat, he kept saying, "I'm curious as to how the others will take it." Somehow I had the feeling that he feared his colleagues would figure out our therapist-patient relationship and react negatively to it. This feeling caused him visible discomfort. For my part, I viewed the situation as a problem that my former patient would have to solve for himself. I was interested in seeing how he would get out of the apparent trap he had obviously set for himself. Without knowing the story of Ali, he used Ali's strategy of being courageous enough to tell the truth. Taking me by the arm, he introduced me to his guests as "Dr. Peseschkian, my psychiatrist."

The people who were there seemed amused. When I thereupon praised the judge for his honesty and openness, some of the guests began to laugh. His news had lost the seriousness it would have had if the same information had gotten around to his colleagues as an open secret. His open admission of psychotherapy had a further result. He joined a self-discovery group for lawyers and judges, and in his office he became a strong advocate of greater use of psychology and psychotherapy in jurisprudential thought.

With Ali's tactics, the judge had sought a solution which at first is a contradiction of logic. According to logic, the judge should have kept quiet about things that would have eventually been detrimental to him. But he would have had to continue to deny his contact with psychotherapy. This tension could have continued indefinitely. His "escape to the front," the courage to tell the truth, enabled him to solve the problem by changing his perspective, *i.e.,* by changing the rules of the game. This produced a surprised reaction from the guests and brought the laughter to the judge's side.

A Reason to Be Thankful

"I need money. Can you lend me a hundred Tuman {Iranian currency}?" a man asked his friend.

"I have the money, but I won't give it to you. Be grateful for that!"

Angrily the friend replied, "That you have money and don't want to give it to me, I can rather understand. But that I should be grateful for it is not only incomprehensible, but a downright disgrace."

"My dear friend," the other answered, "you asked me for money. I could have said, 'Come tomorrow.' Tomorrow I would have said, 'I'm sorry I can't give it to you yet; come back day after tomorrow.' If you had come to me then, I would have said, 'Come at the end of the week.' In this way I could have held you off 'til the end of time, or at least until someone else had given you the money. But you wouldn't have found someone else, because you would have been so preoccupied with coming to me, and you would have always counted on getting my money. So, I tell you in all honesty that I'm not going to give you the money. So, you can look for it elsewhere and try to make your fortune there. Be grateful to me."

A forty-eight-year-old Persian engineer came to me at the advice of his brother, a student in Germany. The man had been suffering from coliclike stomach troubles for six years. He was unable to cite other symptoms. In general it did not seem particularly pleasant for him to be sitting in a psychotherapist's office. He did not talk about his conflicts. Instead, he kept emphasizing the stomach pains that occurred like colic and that had not been successfully treated by medication at home or abroad. In the course of our initial interview, we began to talk about possible sources of conflict: his body, his career and achievements, the future and his fantasies. It seemed that recently the patient had placed his body, particularly his stomach, at the center of all his experiences. I had already observed that in our first meeting. If subjects came up that were in some way conflictual for him, or seemed unpleasant or disturbing, he made a painful grimace and grabbed with his hand for the area of his upper stomach. His greatest concern seemed to be his professional situation. From all appearances, it was determining his conflict. After leaving the university as a certified engineer, he had entered a large firm where he was met with what is generally known as "practice shock." Although well qualified in his field, he did not get along with his colleagues. It wasn't as if open quarrels led to difficulties. On the contrary, the patient was very popular. But a certain uneasiness developed in the engineer himself. If he was given an assignment, he took it on without a mutter. If he was supposed to help a colleague, he did it immediately. If someone needed advice, he was on hand. If someone scolded him, he just smiled. If someone treated him impolitely, unjustly or arbritrarily, he disregarded it. He swallowed insults without dishing them out himself. Even in his own family, he had been the peacemaker and the smoother of conflicts. But, as thankful as his role as confidant and eternal giver was for him, he still suffered inwardly from the cares and burdens that were heaped on him from all sides, burdens which consumed in him with all the patience of a beast of burden.

Our therapeutic dialog did not seem particularly productive. He had identified himself with his role so much that he couldn't distance himself from it. I therefore spoke to him about his concept, his motto. Without thinking about it, and with complete conviction, he quoted Saadi:

If someone causes you sorrow, learn to endure sorrow; through renunciation and forgiveness, you become free from guilt.

This concept contains much of what formed the burdens, the conflict, and the stress under which the patient was suffering: his politeness, the modest suppression of his own interests, his consideration for others, his inability to say no honestly, his guilt feelings, and the fear of rejection, which he obviously wanted to avoid. All of this was crystalized for him in the verse from Saadi. In subsequent conversation, the quote from Saadi proved again and again to be the central point for all his problems in relating to other people. To stimulate a change of perspective, I gave him a counter-concept also from Saadi, which expanded the perspective of his original idea:

110

Two things darken our spirit: silence where one should speak, the speech, where one should be silent.

Going beyond the first concept, the meaning of politeness is expanded to comprise honesty. Our therapy session ended with this expansion of the concept. At the start of the next session, which took place a week later, the patient began on his own to discuss his concept and the prescription of the counter-concept. He also related experiences from his childhood and seemed to have a severe inner dissension, which he described in this way: "I know I'm suffering from it, but I can't just offend the other people."

Here again, he revealed the feelings of guilt and his fears of losing the friendship and esteem of other people, his need to treat all of them correctly, and the denial of the fact that he could not live up to all the responsibilities he had taken on himself. At the end of the session, I prescribed for him the story "A reason to be grateful."

The patient seemed to want to protest against this assignment. He swallowed several times, but, in his well-known polite manner, still said nothing. His reaction came at the next session, like a delayed-action fuse. He complained about me and about psychotherapy, screamed, beat with his fists on the desk, and gestured wildly with his arms. It was behavior I had never before witnessed in him. As if a blockage had been broken up, his aggression and reprimands rattled away at me. It was as if he wanted to see if honesty really worked.

After this emotional outburst, the patient acted very friendly and apologized. He said this had suddenly come over him, and he couldn't do anything about it. But, after his initial surprise, he had been pleased to find that he could express negative feelings without being rejected because of them.

After eight sessions spread out over six weeks—the duration of his stay in Germany—we had worked through his focal problem. In this period of time his symptoms had abated, but kept recurring. It was as if his body still had to complete slowly what the patient had already accomplished in his consciousness and in his experience. In his first letter, six weeks after his return home, he wrote that he had

had no stomach problems the whole time. He said he was able to eat everything and felt much more comfortable at work. This was a successful treatment, a success that continued.

> If I speak unpopular thoughts, it is better than if I say nothing, and am dumb.
>
> (Persian proverb)

The Revenge of the Yes-Man

In the garden of a wise man, there once lived a splendid peacock. The creature was a particular joy for the gardener, who took care of it devotedly. Full of greed and envy, a neighbor kept looking over the fence and couldn't bear the fact that someone had a more beautiful peacock than he. In his envy, he threw rocks at the peacock. The gardener happened to see this and was enraged. But the peacock granted the neighbor no peace. After a while, he began to flatter the gardener by asking if he couldn't at least have a female baby peacock. Categorically the gardener refused. Finally the neighbor turned reverently to the wise master of the house and asked if he couldn't at least have a peacock egg. He wanted to put it under a hen and let her hatch it. The wise man requested that the gardener give the neighbor an egg from the peacock's nest. The gardener did as he was told. After a while the neighbor came and complained to the wise man, "Something is wrong with the egg. My chickens sat on it for weeks, but no peacock wants to slip out of it." Angrily he went back home. The wise man called to his gardener, "You gave our neighbor an egg. Why doesn't a peacock hatch from it?" The gardener replied, "I cooked the egg first." The wise man looked at him in astonishment. Then the gardener said in an apologetic tone, "You told me I should give him a peacock egg. But you didn't say whether it should be cooked or not. . . ."

With or against their will, the social connections between people are formed by one order or by many orders. Social partners can take on equal roles within a large sphere, or they can be structured from top to bottom, that is, divided into upper order or lower order. People like to circumscribe these relationships with concepts like authority, obedience, discipline.

Along with the question of whether and how a certain relationship to authority is justified, it is important to ask how we react to it. Aside from unconditional submission and anti-authoritarian revolt described in psychoanalysis as symbolic murder of one's father, there are countless other possible reactions. They are distinguished by their intensity and the type of authority crisis. The question is, which of the two poles—submission or rejection—is in the foreground. Even if we only see that the one person reacts adaptively and obediently, and the other defiantly and anti-authoritarianly, this conduct is also a reaction to an acute or biographical conflict. Where disobedience and resistance character-ize a person's behavior, there is quite often a need for an absolute authority that one can trust. On the other hand, there are many people who seem obedient and adaptive, but are really in the midst of a latent, silent crisis of authority, a strong inner revolt, which is often noticeable only in strange ways.

The twenty-one-year-old merchant Peter S., who worked in his father's shop, described his problem in this way:

"For some time now, I have been feeling less and less capable of taking on responsibilities. I have a lot of trouble dealing with the demands of my work, because I tire easily. My ability to concentrate has also diminished a great deal. Then I am dissatisfied with myself and have a tendency to act aggressively toward others. My father often reproaches me. Outwardly I have accepted these rebukes with indifference and stoic quiet, but inwardly I have felt a negative attitude toward my parents. As far as physical complaints are concerned, I have had headaches with increasing frequency. Most of the time I feel quite tired and feel I can hardly accomplish anything anymore. I try to disguise my weaknesses with all sorts of trickery, even though I don't feel relieved by doing this." (Excerpts from the initial interview)

The patient's obedience expressed itself in extraordinary politeness, which could be viewed as a way of inhibiting the exertion of his own will and as a result of his father's dominating authority. The father's demands on his son had absolute authority; at least, this is how the patient experienced it. He accepted all the business tasks his father delegated to him, even if they were too

113

much for him. "Cheating" provided the only escape. He caused business letters he couldn't answer to disappear, "forgot" to make a note of important phone calls, and neglected to carry on with assignments and customer orders. His only excuse for his professional shortcomings was, "I'm simply overburdened with work. It's too much for me. I'm not suited for this profession."

This opinion would have actually called more for professional training than for psychotherapeutic treatment. But the fact was that the patient had sought therapy on his own. He obviously needed help with his conflicts and did not think a change of careers would be a real solution. In fact, he believed that would have just been an escape. He was not yet conscious of this chain of thoughts when he started therapy. It would not even have been comprehensible to him at that time without some preparation. I thus told him the story of the peacock egg and the neighbor. By then we had reached the end of our third session and had established a relaxed and friendly atmosphere. I told him that particular story because of its treatment of authority and how one can deal with it.

Peter S. made a face and smiled: "My father tells me I should take care of a certain letter or phone call. I do it then, and in my own way, of course. As far as I'm concerned, the letter or the call is then a finished matter. And I've escaped my father once again. That's what's so funny about all this. I really do like my career, but, when I get an assignment or order from my father, it's as if I'm locked. I shift my motor into neutral, and it doesn't move forward even a centimeter."

Therapist: "Does your father also realize the meaning of your carelessness?"

Peter S.: "I don't think so. He simply thinks I'm unreliable, messy, sloppy, lazy, and perhaps even stupid. But that I'm going against his authority—that's something he's probably not caught on to. I say yes and amen to everything, even when it irks me. Most of all I get angry that he gives me directions without any consideration."

We worked through the actual conflict in a systematic way, under the aspect of the problem "politeness-honesty." This problem had led the father's demand for obedience to become a conflict for

114

the patient. The counter-concept to his passive resistance was active resistance: "Say what can't be done and explain why not." In this way, the conflict was raised from the inadequate realm of childish defiance and was placed into the area of a concrete argument, which the patient could more easily control. This also gave the patient the feeling that he had not been arbitrarily placed in his father's control; he could also express his own wishes and needs without fear of punishment. At the same time, we also worked through the basic conflict and the life history of this conflict, so that he learned to understand why he had adopted this defensive-masochistic attitude in dealing with his father. He also came to realize what obstacles stood in the way of honesty and openness.

A Good Model

A mullah wanted to protect his daughter from the dangers of life. When the time had come and she had grown into a true flower of beauty, he took her aside and told her about the baseness and malice of the world. "My dear daughter," he said, "remember what I tell you. All men want only one thing. Men are cunning. They set traps wherever they can. You don't realize how you sink deeper and deeper into the swamp of their desires. I want to show you the way of unhappiness. First the man swoons about your best features, and he admires you. Then he invites you to go out with him. Then the two of you pass his house, and he mentions that he just wants to fetch his coat. He asks you if you wouldn't like to come in the house with him. Upstairs he invites you to have a seat, and he offers you some tea. The two of you listen to music, and, when the time is right, he suddenly throws himself on you. In this way you are violated, and we are violated, your mother and I. Our family is violated, and our good reputation is gone."

The daughter took these words of her father to heart. Some time later she came up to her father and smiled proudly. "Dad," she asked, "are you a prophet? How did you know how everything happens? It was just as you described it. First he admired my beauty. Then he asked me out. As if by coincidence we passed his house. There the poor fellow noticed he had forgotten his coat. And, so I wouldn't be alone, he invited me to come on into his apartment. As good manners require, he offered me tea and brightened the day with beautiful music. At that point, I thought of your words and I knew exactly what would happen. But you see, I am worthy to be your daughter. When I felt the moment coming, I threw myself on him and violated him, his parents, his family, his good reputation, and his esteem!"

A forty-eight-year-old merchant come to me because of a magazine article about my book *Positive Psychotherapy.* His problem basically dealt with concepts like authority crises, the generation gap, conflicts of self-esteem, moral scruples, and so forth. He claimed he wasn't coming because of himself, but because of his daughter, who was causing him much grief. After graduating from school, his daughter Susanna had immediately moved to another city so that she could attend the university. He had not at all agreed with this idea and could still not accept the fact that Susi, as he sweetly called her, now lived, defenseless, in a strange city.

His complaint always arrived at the same point, namely, that he was in a much better position to protect his daughter from harm. "I've had a lot of experiences in my life, including bad ones," he said. "The young people today are so carefree and unconstrained and never think of the consequences. You know, don't you, where there are dangers lurking. If my daughter could judge things according to my experiences, she could save herself and us a lot of sorrow and aggravation." The patient had traveled from the Ruhr district for an individual intervention treatment. The therapeutic efforts therefore had to be focused on a few central areas. Even the patient's compulsive traits had to initially be disregarded. Through his overprotectiveness, the patient tried to banish all threatening dangers and to avoid all the threatening things that would have come back upon him if his concepts had been called into question. Without a doubt, he had considerable sexual-aggressive wishes, which were nevertheless repressed and would have required longer treatment. In the meantime, they could not be part of his consciousness; in the intervention treatment, I thus had to use other means. I told him, the overly concerned and inwardly overburdened father, the story "A Good Model."

At first the patient had listened with great interest. At the end of the story, he made an almost shocked face and soon thereafter began to laugh. I had the impression that he identified with the mullah and that the sudden change of perspective had surprised him as much as it had the hero of the story. Without my asking, he suddenly told about his family situation and mentioned how he had suffered under the authority of his father. "If I say water runs up the mountain, then water runs up the mountain." This had been the father's attitude. Through the story and its transference to his situation, the ambiguity of his overprotective attitude became clear. He was able to see the generation task he had unconsciously tried to fulfill: the task of maintaining the line of descent for authority within the family; of transferring his wishes to his children; of demanding obedience even from his adult daughter; and of preventing the independence that would have meant for him the discharge of his parental duties.

We dealt with these ideas in our following conversation. It seemed as if the patient had set out on a voyage of discovery, for he was always so surprised when he was able to see previously unknown connections. All of this, of course, was still a far cry from being a complete treatment, but he was able to come to terms with his conflict and its consequences for the relationship with his daughter. In a letter, he wrote to me that he was still preoccupied with the story and the themes it presented, and that he had become much more critical of himself.

The Woolen Beard

In a fabric and yarn shop at the bazaar, a woman searched long and carefully for some wool cloth because she wanted to make her husband, an ahaa, a cloak. She was concerned most of all that the fabric be made of pure sheep's wool and nothing else. "Take this wonderful fabric," the merchant said as he praised the qualitites of a bolt of cloth. "Your husband will feel so good in this, he'll think he's being carried by the angels into paradise." These words caused the woman's resolve to weaken. She wanted to be sure of just one thing. "Can you swear that this is made of pure wool?" she asked the merchant. "Of course," he replied, "I swear by all the prophets, that this," and with these words he drew his hand from the cloth and began stroking his long white beard, "is made of nothing but pure wool."

"I can't believe anything my husband says any more. He twists everything the way he wants it." These words were spoken by a forty-five-year-old German woman, a physician married to a Persian doctor. Her complaint always ended with her telling about a frequently occurring experience: Her husband often left the house with his guests, mostly fellow-countrymen. He usually accompanied them somewhere, such as to the train station, and stayed away for several hours. "And when he does that, he always says he'll come right back." The patient was very bitter about this. In her complaints, one could also hear an indictment against the "Eastern way of life," to which the patient attributed her husband's problems. I gave her the story of the wool beard and asked that she read it.

The story caused her to smile. "Although my husband is a doctor, he could have just as easily been the fabric merchant. But I'm not like that. When I say something, for me it has obvious validity." With these words, we were already in the disentanglement of the transcultural problem. The story of the wool beard had helped the woman get a better understanding of her husband's mentality.

Expensive Frugality

A man came before the judge because of bribery. Since everything pointed to the man's guilt, all that was left was for the judge to pronounce judgment. The judge was a reasonable man. He offered the man three choices from which he could select his punishment. The accused was supposed either to pay a hundred tuman, or to be whipped fifty times, or else to eat five kilos of onions. "That's certainly won't be so hard," the man thought as he bit into the first onion. But after he'd eaten exactly three quarters of a pound of raw onions, he was overcome by repulsion as he looked at these fruits of the field. His eyes began to water and streams of tears poured down his cheeks. "High court," he cried, "spare me the onions. I'd rather take the fifty lashes." In his thoughts he believed he would cunningly be able to save his money. After all, he was famous for his greed. The bailiff undressed him and placed him on the bench. But the sight of the powerful bailiff and the plaint rod caused him to tremble. With every blow to his back, he screamed louder until, with the tenth blow, he finally wailed, "Great Ghazi, have pity on me. Spare me these blows." The judge shook his head. Then the man, who had wanted to avoid the blows and wanted to keep his money, ended up sampling all three punishments, begged, "Just let me pay the hundred tuman."

A forty-two-year-old patient became increasingly defensive in his therapeutic treatment. He cancelled sessions, but kept coming anyway because of his ailments. These were mostly anxiety and depression. Already in taking the inventory for differentiation analysis, I was struck by the fact that he was very frugal with money, did without services that cost money, and did not invite guests to his house because "it's too expensive and doesn't produce anything." As defense for missing some of our meetings, he would say, "I had too much to do, I forgot the appointment," and so forth.

At the moment when the subject of frugality came up, the spell seemed to be broken. His words spewed forth. "I've been putting up with this for a long time. I pay far more for psychotherapy than I do for my family doctor. I've been going to him for treatment for eight years. I can't afford to pay so much for psychotherapy. . . ." The patient did something very important for psychotherapy: He talked about what was bothering him.

At first glance, his arguments seemed so convincing that one could have considered terminating the treatment. But on the other hand, the financial question was not the core of the argumentation. The patient had enough money at his disposal. And, even if he hadn't, there would have been ways to ease the expense. His criticism seemed to be a symptom that concerned psychotherapy as well as his own conflict. His valuation of frugality and the expenditure of money represented a basic conflict that had led to existential insecurity and social isolation. It was now my task to counter his resistance to the problem of frugality. This resistance was at first the actual theme of the session. The patient repeated his

119

criticism in a stereotyped manner and did not seem ready for any progress. His notion of frugality controlled him so much that he was no longer capable of having new thoughts of his own. The patient got himself out of his dead end with the help of the Persian story "Expensive frugality." The story provided him some temporary identification but still gave him enough distance to think about his own situation in the framework of the story. The patient was silent for a while and put a lot of effort into his thoughts about it. Finally he said, "I think the story actually has to do with me. What have I sacrificed for my health during all this time: visits to spas, special medication, books about health, and so on? Now I've started psychotherapy and have some confidence and feel that you understand me and psychotherapy can help me. Now I suddenly want to save money with the therapy. It occurs to me that I have often denied myself real possibilities because of my damned frugality. And afterwards I still have to pay." From this point on, the constructive entry into the conflict-laden norm—frugality—was possible.

Just as there might be a resistance to the cost of therapy, problems can develop because the patient suddenly does not have enough time for it. This resistance can be based on the fact that, in his time plan, the patient actually sees little possibility for psychotherapy, and that he regards it as less important than other interests. From this, one could conclude that there is a lack of motivation, but sometimes this conclusion proves to be short-sighted. Through his decision, the patient adopts an evaluation that has certain stipulations and must therefore be investigated. The patient's daily schedule can provide information as to whether he really has time or not, and why he gives priority to other interests. Lack of time might be a defense against psychotherapy and represent a rationalization for the patient and the therapist. One senses that the therapy is endangered to the extent that one would rather not go into it further. Even this motive has background factors that are usually not accessible to the patient. He carries around his shortage of time like a protective wall.

A patient suffering from severe heart ailments, vegetatively functional disorders and anxiety, claimed after the initial interview that he did not have time for psychotherapy. A further delay in the treatment would have probably lead to a worsening of his complaints. Even this argument, however, could not persuade the patient. For him, the actualizing capability "time" was more important to him than a continuation of the treatment.

In his background information, I was struck by the fact that the patient had to sacrifice a lot of time when his symptoms occurred, all in spite of his alleged lack of time. At such times, he stayed in bed for several days. As an achievement-oriented person, he was confronted by the concept "Time is money." As a contrast to this, I quoted a saying by Lichtenberg, "The people who never have time do the least." Here I used a proverb instead of an Eastern story. The patient understood the concept immediately. Whereas he had previously refused all efforts at establishing communication, he now began to discuss his problem, one that was centralized around the actualizing capabilities—achievement and time.

The Secret of the Long Beard

A scholar well known for his knowledge and his magnificently long white beard walked through the alleys of Shiraz one evening. Lost in thought, he came upon a throng of water-carriers who made fun of him. The boldest in the group finally stepped forward, bowed deeply, and said, "Great master, my comrades and I have made a bet. Please tell us, where does your beard lie when you sleep at night? On the bedspread, or under it?" The scholar, aroused from his thoughts, looked up in amazement and answered kindly, "I don't know myself. I've never thought about it. I'll check into it. Expect me here tomorrow at the same time. I will tell you then."

When night had come and the scholar had gone to bed, he found that he couldn't get to sleep. With wrinkled brow, he thought about where he kept his beard. On the bedspread? Under it? As much as he thought about it, his memory could give him no answer. Finally he decided to run an experiment. He put his beard on top of the spread and wanted to fall asleep. But inner unrest seized his heart. Was this really the right position? If it was right, then why hadn't he fallen asleep a long time ago? With this in mind, he pulled his beard under the covers. But this did little good. Sleep was far away as ever. "It can't have been this way," he concluded, and again put the beard on top of the bedspread.

In this way he struggled through the whole night—first with the beard on the bed, then under the spread—without a moment's sleep as the answer to his question. The next evening he approached the young water carrier. "My friend," he said, "I used to sleep with this glorious beard of mine, and I could enjoy the sweetest slumber every time. But, since you questioned me, I can't sleep anymore. An answer to your question is impossible, and my beard, the crowing glory of my wsidom and the sign of my noble age, has become strange to me. I don't know if I can ever again feel comfortable with it."

A forty-one-year-old technician had come for treatment because of compulsive acts and thoughts. He had already been treated twice at a psychiatric-psychotherapeutic clinic.

"I can't take it any longer. I can't sleep. . . . If something changes around me, I simply fall apart. Everything has to have the order that I'm used to. I myself have the feeling that it is strange, but I can't sleep if my wife has just changed the bed linens. I have to get up and put the old ones on again. My wife has already declared I'm completely crazy. I certainly don't want that, but that's the way it goes."

As the patient recalled, his father had been extremely exact and conscientious and could tolerate no disorderliness. If his room was not straightened up, he had had to go to bed as early as 7:00 P.M. There he had indulged in fantasies and had imagined how he could take revenge on his father. At one session the patient seemed completely desperate. With an unusually pathetic voice, he reported, "I am totally crazy. I can't even drive a car anymore. Last week I accidentally changed the position of the driver's seat, and now I don't know where it should be. I push it back and forth, but it never seems right. I've never before felt so unsafe in a car." For this patient, the experience of compulsion stood in the foreground. It completely occupied his consciousness. The direct goal of our therapeutic dialog was to create a certain distance to his compulsion. This is why I told him the story "The Secret of the Long

Beard." Unexpectedly the patient began to laugh and immediately related the story to himself: "That fellow has the same problem I do. He doesn't have an easy time of it, even if he is a wise man." In one of the following sessions, the patient told me that he had had to think about the man many times. To his astonishment, driving a car had suddenly become easy for him again. "I've thought a lot about it: sitting forward or sitting back is just like having the beard above or below." With the aid of the story, the patient was able to imagine a scene comparable to his own situation and which offered him obvious help, at least in terms of driving a car.

A Man, a Word

After hearing an enthusiastic and youthful sermon from the mullah, a friend asked him, "Mullah, most honored one, how old are you?" The mullah looked at the younger interrogator and replied, "I have dried more shirts in the sun than you. My age is no secret. I'm forty years old."

About twenty years later the two met again. The mullah had gray hair, and his beard looked as if it had been sprinkled with flour. "Mullah, most honored one," the friend began, "I haven't seen you for a long time. How old are you now?"

The mullah answered, "You curious man, you want to know everything. I'm forty."

Astonished, the friend asked, "How is it that you gave the same answer when I asked you twenty years ago? That can't be right."

Angrily, the mullah responded, "Why shouldn't that be right? What do I care about twenty years? At that time I told you I'm forty, and I still say that. For me one thing is important: a man—a word."

Society in general and the group in which one lives are dependent on time. Demands and expectations can change (process of increase, urbanization, differentiation). This change in the environment is not without consequences for the people living in it. The role expectations imposed on people, and which they set for themselves, can change with the needs of the surroundings.

The changes and developments that a person experiences take

place against the background of historical, cultural, and social events. Psychotherapy, however, deals less with the general theme than with the individual's ability to change. The word "conformity" is suspect in today's world, and ought to be replaced with a term such as the "ability to adjust to change." This ability to adapt is an essential condition for treatment. I'd like to explain what I mean by using an example from internal medicine and endocrinology.

A particular patient suffering from an overactive thyroid could run around in shirtsleeves even in cold weather. While others froze, he felt comfortable. The physical explanation for this was that, with the overactive thyroid, the man's metabolism was also speeded up and the body produced excessive heat. The patient suffered especially during the heat of the summer. His suffering expressed itself in difficulties with adaptation. While the body of the healthy person can adjust to wide ranges of temperature, this ability was considerably limited for the patient. He was more susceptible to the temperature changes in his environment.

The situation of a neurotic patient has much to do with this kind of adaptive difficulty. With him it is not the temperature difference that causes problems, but rather changes of behavior and expectations in the social world. Hence, a person suffering from compulsiveness, a person who considers orderliness to be the crucial factor in life, will have trouble adjusting to any kind of fluctuations in his system of order. In a certain realm of order, the compulsive patient is highly differentiated. When this realm is overstepped and other ideas of order come into play, the person's ability to adjust, his flexibility, is placed under too much stress. He cannot deal with the new situation. He responds to it with anxiety, panic, aggression, or physical complaints. As was said by a thirty-nine-year-old woman with coronary and circulatory problems, chronic constipation, and sleep disorders, "If I haven't cleaned up my room, it means 'I don't love you any more.' That used to cause me to panic. Today I am more than pedantic, and this gets me into a lot of conflict with my husband and children." A thirty-five-year-old economist said, "I learned to do one thing after another. Everything has to have its sequence. First comes brushing my teeth, then washing up; then I shave, get all dressed up, sit down at the breakfast table, drink two cups of coffee, read the paper, and then go to the toilet. If this sequence is disrupted I completely fall apart; I have trouble with my bowel movements, and the whole day is a loss."

A fixed attitude like this can be called into question during a time of crisis. But just changing one's opinion does not produce a complete change. In most cases, an emotional crisis brings along a strong affective involvement, inner doubts, disappointments, and a loss of courage.

Changing one's opinion back and forth, even just a temporary lack of orientation, is so frightening for some people that they choose the other extreme. To protect themselves from doubts or, better said, desperation, they flee into a rigidity that they then regard as loyalty and firmness of character. In order not to have to change their behavior, they may disregard information that could increase their doubts.

The Servant of the Eggplant

A mighty ruler in the ancient East liked to eat bademdjan, eggplant. He couldn't get enough of it, and even had a servant whose only task involved preparing the eggplant in as tasty a way as possible. The ruler raved about it. "How fabulous this vegetable is," he exclaimed, "How divine it tastes. How elegant it looks. Eggplant is the best thing on earth."

"You are certainly right," the servant replied.

That very day, the ruler greedily ate so much eggplant that he became ill. He felt as if his stomach would turn upside down, and it seemed that all the eggplant he had ever eaten now wanted again to see the light of day. He moaned, "No more eggplant. I don't want to ever again see this food of hell. Just the thought of it makes me ill. Eggplant is the most horrible vegetable I know."

"You're certainly right," replied the servant.

The ruler was startled to hear this. "Today, when I was still talking about how magnificent the eggplant is, you agreed with me. Now that I'm talking about how terrible it is, you again agree with me. How do you explain that?" "My lord," said the servant, "I am your servant, not the servant of the eggplant."

The servant is clever. He knows the role he must play at the court. He knows which authorities and dangers are tied to it, and he conducts himself so that his own interests are not slighted. He does not point out the ruler's lack of logic, nor does he play the role of advocate for the eggplant. His conduct is pragmatic and goal-oriented. Many people, of course, might criticize him for lacking personal involvement.

A twenty-seven-year-old employee began psychotherapy more by accident than by design. Bothered by stomach problems, he had been told by his family doctor that psychological issues might be the root of the trouble. At an early stage of his therapy, he began to talk about his career, especially his problems with his boss. Whenever he had developed his own ideas on a new project, his boss rejected them. "He does what he wants, but I can't do anything," the patient commented. And he really did everything he could. Even in his free time, he worked until late at night, developing new models. But each morning he discovered that his ideas were not only unwanted, but were also looked upon as a nuisance. For the patient, who placed a lot of importance on achievement and professional success, the situation at work became more and more unbearable. Since he could not react openly, he reacted with his body. His stomach pains were a protest against his boss's injustice.

We won't go into the basic conflict and the psychodynamics here. But it is important that we examine the direct crisis intervention, which had as its main goal the reduction of the patient's suffering. The professional involvement and patient's ambition were not the sources of conflict; nor was the problem his need to be effective in the company and to carry through with his ideas. For the patient's therapy, two things were important: the expectant attitude, which he kept hidden behind diverse activities, and his inability to take into consideration the psychological situation of his authoritative, paternalistic boss. In this connection, the story, "The servant of the eggplant," provided the patient with

126

a counter-concept. It was not a model, but a stimulus for him to become more aware of his own typical reactions, to see them in a more differentiated way, and to come to terms with them.

The Glass Sarcophagus

An Eastern king had an enchanting wife whom he loved more than anything. Her beauty illuminated his life. Whenever he had time, he tried to be with her. One day she suddenly died, and the king was left alone in great sorrow. "Never, never will I leave my beloved young wife," he cried out, "even if death has taken every bit of life fom her beautiful features." He put his wife into a glass sarcophagus in the largest room of the palace, and put his bed next to it so he wouldn't be separated from her even for a minute. This closeness to his departed wife was his sole comfort; it alone gave him peace.

But it was a hot summer. Despite the coolness of the palace, the woman's body slowly began to decompose. Soon beads of sweat formed on the woman's noble brow. Her lovely face changed its color and became more bloated from one day to the next. But in his great love the king did not notice this. Soon the sweetish smell of decay filled the whole room, and no servant dared even stick his nose beyond the door. The king himself, with heavy heart, took his bed and carried it into the next room. Although the windows were all wide open, the odor of transitoriness followed him. No attar of roses was strong enough to conceal it. Finally he took his green sash, the sign of his royalty, and tied it over his nose. But nothing seemed to help. All his servants and friends abandoned him. The only ones who still kept company with him were the huge black flies that hummed around him.

Then the king lost consciousness. The hakim, the physician, had him brought into the palatial garden. When the king woke up, a fresh breeze was blowing over him. The fragrance of the flowers gently aroused his senses, and the gurgling of the fountains was like music to his ears. It seemed to him as if his beloved were still alive. After a few days the king was again filled with health and life. Contemplative, he looked into the center of a rose and suddenly remembered how beautiful his wife had been when she was alive, and how more and more horrible her corpse had become

127

from day to day. He broke off the rose, placed it on the sarcophagus and
ordered his servants to bury the body.

(Persian Story)

A forty-four-year-old female skilled laborer had come for an initial interview at the request of her family doctor. She was suffering from abnormal grief. It was the beginning of a treatment that went on for twenty sessions and represented a difficult struggle for me as well as for the patient. To illustrate her situation, I will present some excerpts from the first interview.

"I'm at the brink of despair when I try to realize that my husband, who was once healthy and normal, suddenly became so mentally ill that he committed suicide. Along with the overwhelming pain, I reproach myself for being so hard on him during our eleven years of marriage. I nagged him a lot and screamed at him for a lot of little things. I am convinced that a more even-tempered and happy wife could have prevented his illness or at least kept it from being so serious.

"Along with the pain, there is also pity, pity for my husband, who had to die so young. This pity is almost worse than the pain I feel at his loss, and I must admit that I've often thought of killing myself. The only thing that has kept me from it is the fact that I feel responsible toward my aging mother."

At the start of the therapy she kept saying, "Isn't it possible that my behavior made my husband sick and caused him to kill himself?" Regardless of what time it was, she would call me up to ask this question again.

Similarly, I discovered that she talked about her problems with her family doctor, her neighbors, and all the people she had previously had contact with. The result of this obtrusive cry for help was that all her friends felt put upon by her. She became more and more isolated with her problems. A rational, logical conversation seemed impossible. The patient knew everything better and refused every insight except her self-recriminations and stereotyped admissions of guilt. All of this pointed to an unfavorable prognosis. But, step by step, we reduced her compulsions. Instead of continually dealing with the patient's compulsively

128

depressed concepts, I tried to help her differentiate the image of her husband that she had built up over the course of time. This caused her difficulty. She raved about the idealized positive qualities of her deceased husband, but at the moment when negative subjects were raised, she pulled back. To prevent the surfacing of any forbidden aggressions against her departed husband, she replaced his short-comings with her own insufficiencies and admissions of guilt. "I didn't give him enough money," she confessed, "I told him I deserved more. For a long time I refused to have sex with him. I was insensitive to his needs," and so forth. And then, to make these utterances less sharp, she always added, "I really didn't mean to do what I did. I always apologized right away. I asked him not to be angry."

At that point I gave her the following story to read.

About the Crow and the Peacock

In the palace park, a black crow perched on the branches of an orange tree. Down on the well-tended lawn, a peacock marched around proudly. The crow screeched, "How can one even permit such a strange bird to enter this park? He walks around as arrogantly as if he were the sultan himself. And with those downright ugly feet! And his feathers such a horrible shade of blue! I would never wear a color like that. He drags his tail around like a fox." The crow stopped and waited silently for a reply. The peacock did not say anything for a while, but then he began to speak with a melancholy smile, "I don't think your assertions correspond to reality. The bad things you say about me rest on misunderstandings. You say I'm arrogant, because I hold my head up so that my shoulder feathers stick out and a double chin disfigures my neck. In reality I'm anything but arrogant. I know my ugly features, and I know my feet are wrinkled and like leather. This actually bothers me so much that I hold my head erect in order not to see my ugly feet. You see only my ugly parts. You close your eyes to my fine points and to my beauty. Haven't you noticed that? What you call ugly is exactly what people admire in me."

(After P. Etessami)

For the patient, this story became an example by which she oriented herself. She remarked that she had denied her husband's mistakes, areas of conflicts, and sensitive areas just as the crow had disregarded the peacock's positive features. In a letter that she sent to me during this phase of the treatment, she wrote, "Actually I have given preference to my negative side rather than to the positive. It is my misfortune that I have such a good memory as far as the past is concerned. I still have problems in seeing my husband's negative side. And I wasn't really so bad either." These thoughts were the starting point from which we were able to bring the patient out of the vicious circle she had found herself in.

From the compulsive repetition of long-past conflicts and self-recriminations we moved on to a new stage of the treatment. The patient spoke of her own past, her relationship to her parents, and the expectations she had had of her husband. There had developed a mother-daughter relationship in which the patient, despite her professional successes, still played the role of the helpless little child. The husband's role was determined by this mother-daughter unit. He was an intruder, and both woman demanded that he agree to their ideas of frugality, orderliness, sexuality, and contact. Nevertheless, open confrontations occurred rarely. The patient often played the role of plaintiff. Her husband, to whom she appeared to attribute great powers of resistance, was, according to her, weak and submissive. Conflicts were subconsciously answered by appealing to her readiness to admit guilt. This worked well with the patient's mechanism for dealing with conflict.

After we had intensively worked through the inventory stage, after the stage of denial had been overcome, and after the patient had become more aware of her guilt feelings and their causes, she began to verbalize her own needs and interests and to expand her goals. Despite these obvious signs of progress, which had at first seemed impossible, the patient occasionally fell back into nostalgically idealizing her departed husband. Her separation from objects that had been dear to him almost brought about a new case of mourning for her. She reacted to it with guilt feelings, anxieties and inner dissolution.

During one session, she began talking about these difficulties.

She toyed with the idea of giving away some of her husband's furniture that she had previously hated. But she said she just couldn't bring herself to do it. At this point, I told her the story of the glass sarcophagus. At first the patient was struck by the story. The description of the decaying body made a deep impression on her. The story reminded her of aggressions she had previously been unable to admit: aggressions that found expression in the images of decay and in the act of separation. Because of her upbringing and relationship with her mother, she had been bound to the idea that dissolution was negative and would be punished. By means of this story, she was told indirectly that dissolution can be good for achieving something new.

No Master Falls from the Sky

A magician was performing his art before the sultan and winning the enthusiasm of his audience. The sultan himself was filled with admiration and exclaimed, "God, help me, what a miracle, what a genie!"

But his vizier gave him pause for thought as he said, "Your highness, no master falls from the sky. The magician's art is the result of his industriousness and his practice."

The sultan wrinkled his brow. His vizier's disagreement had spoiled his pleasure in the magic acts. "You ungrateful man! How can you claim that such skill comes from practice? It is just as I said: either you have talent or you don't." He looked at the vizier contemptuously and cried, "You don't have any talent anyway—away with you to the dungeon. There you can ponder my words. And so you won't be lonely, and so you will have one of your kind right there, you will have a calf as a cellmate."

Starting on his first day in the cell, the vizier practiced picking up the calf and carrying it up the steps of the dungeon tower. Months went by. The calf grew into a powerful steer, and, with each day of practice, the vizier's power increased.

One day, the sultan remembered the man in the cell. He had him brought to him. When he saw him, he was overcome with amazement. "God help me, what a miracle, what a genie."

The vizier, carrying the steer on outstretched arms, answered with the

131

same words as the other time: "Your highness, no master falls from the sky.
In your mercy you gave me this animal. My strength is the result of my
industriousness and my practice."

In the magician, the king wants to see someone who has a unique and excellent skill that no one else has achieved. He removes the magician's achievements from their connections in reality and idealizes him.

It is said: Either you can make contact with people, or you can't. Either we have the ability to circumvent our problems, or we don't. Either you have luck going for you, or you don't. This definite "either-or" is behind the idea that one is born with certain abilities, or else he doesn't have them at all. In our story, the vizier counters this either-or with a third possibility. For him, the magician's art is the result of his industriousness and practice. In this way, the either-or is replaced by the idea that a person can basically achieve everything if he simply has enough time at his disposal and is ready to use his time to achieve his goals. The vizier proves this assumption through his own example.

In a family therapy case, the treatment had gone so far that the original patient, under psychotherapeutic supervision, could be appointed as "therapist" in his own environment. The patient, a thirty-eight-year-old employee, suffered primarily from the idea that he was less capable of accomplishing something, less creative, and less independent than other people. His thirty-two-year-old wife had made him even more certain that this was the case. Her motto was, "See what the others have done. You'll never do that." This sentence, "You'll never do that" had accompanied the patient almost his entire life. He told me, "My mother always admired boys who had accomplished something, who had finished school and gone to college. Those were the models that were always held up for me. They were models that I couldn't approach."

The patient was interested in art, especially painting. Along with his wife, he went to exhibitions and admired the artists, but had never tried painting himself. During therapy, he developed the initiative to pick up a brush and enroll in a painting course. His wife didn't like this idea. She said to him, "You should leave painting to the professionals. You aren't a genius." But the patient didn't let this discourage him. In fact, after his first successes, he inspired her to try her hand at charcoal drawing.

About six months later, during a checkup, his wife said, "I had no idea of the talents that are in a person. My husband paints in a way that appeals to me a lot. We used to have copies of Chagall, Franz Marc, and Picasso in our living room, but we replaced them with original paintings by my husband. He also had a picture framed that I painted. I think the experiment with art has given both of us self-confidence and has stimulated us to be more experimental in other things as well."

It seems impossible to us that everyone can do everything. But that is not the issue. The important thing is that we are able to develop a multitude of talents if we give them space and time to develop.

You Are Omniscient!

It is told that an adherent of an Islamic sect once came to his sheik, the leader of his religious community, famous as a fortuneteller and clairvoyant. The man said, "O sheik, my wife is pregnant. I'm afraid she will give birth to a daughter. I beg of you, please pray that God, in his mercy, give me a son."

The sheik replied, "Go get some wonderful melons, bread, and cheese so that my throng of believers, once satisfied, can utter the prayer for you."

"By the light of my eyes I'll do it," the man said. He then went and got everything the sheik had ordered.

After the meal, the throng prayed, and even the sheik lowered himself to say a few words. "Be certain," the sheik spoke, "you will have a son, and, when he is ten years old, he will enter our order."

His wife, however, gave birth to a daughter who, moreover, was very ugly. The man was very sad about this and came to the sheik and complained, "Your prayers did not bring what you had promised. You said I'd have a son. Now I have a daughter, and an ugly one at that."

To this the sheik replied, "The food that you brought me at that time was surely not prepared in true faith and with purity of intention. If you

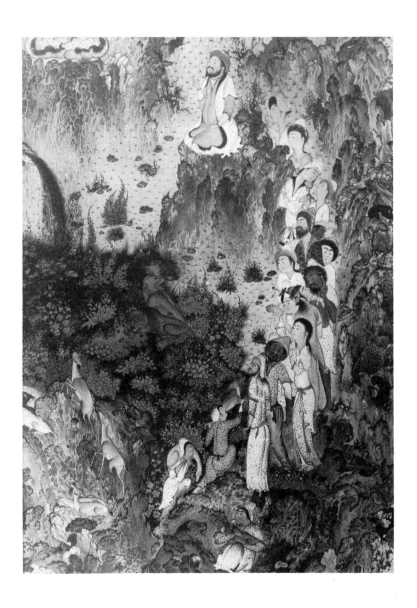

had done it with pure intent and with all your heart, I swear to you that you would have had a son. But, even though the child is a girl, be assured that she will bring you more joy and more gain than a son. For, in my vision, I saw your daughter as a celebrated scholar." Consoled by these words, the man went away.

Two months later the daughter died. The man again went to the sheik and said, "O sheik, my daughter has died. I must say that your prayer had no effect whatsoever."

The sheik replied, "I told you your daughter would bring you more gain than a son. Had your daughter lived, her heart would have been crushed by all the ugliness of this world. So it was good that she died."

When the sheik had said this, a throng of followers jumped up and threw themselves at his feet. And they all sang. "Inshallah Taallah. We hope the strength of health will always be with you. We will always be your humble servants. Indeed, you are omniscient. Your breath has living power and your being is not less than that of the prophets!"

(After Sheik Behai)

Where concepts do not agree with reality, reality is frequently made to conform to the concept. This form of resistance and inner opposition proves to be very tenacious, often almost invincible. One is inclined to say, "I can't have made a mistake. What my parents told me is and remains true. What my doctor says is right. You can say what you want, but I am right."

This game of being right can be extended to everything: to education, marriage, profession, science, politics, religion. The concept itself is shielded from reality in that reality is considered impossible, or is reinterpreted according to that concept. This reaction shows that, in the realm of human relationships, there is not one reality, but many realities which we perceive through the filter of our concepts and attitudes. It becomes critical when the concepts are removed from every check that reality could provide; the concepts then become ends in themselves. In this case, communication loses its character of mutuality. A patient described it this way: "It's like throwing stones against a rubber wall. The stones keep coming back."

In a similar way, patients and many of our fellow-men juggle their concepts. One can hardly deal with them through argument; sometimes this is entirely impossible. These people have an answer for everything that counters their ideas.

I'm Just as Strong as Forty Years Ago

Three old men, all good friends, sat together and talked about the joys of youth and the burdens of old age. "Ah," moaned the one, "my limbs don't want to do what I want them to. How I used to run like a greyhound, and now my legs leave me in the lurch so much, I can hardly place one foot in front of the other."

"You're right," the second man assured him. "I have the feeling my youthful powers have seeped away like water in the desert. The times have changed, and between the millstones of time we've changed, too."

The third, a mullah, a lay preacher, hardly less rickety than his comrades, shook his head and said, "I don't understand you fellows. What you are complaining about, I haven't experienced in myself. I'm just as strong as I was forty years ago." But the other two couldn't believe this. "Sure, sure," protested the mullah. "And I just had proof of it yesterday. For as long as I can remember, I've had a big heavy oak chest in my bedroom. Forty years ago I tried to lift it, but would you believe, old friends, what happened? I couldn't lift it. Yesterday the idea occurred to me to try lifting it again. I tried it with all my might, but again I was unable to do it. But it proves one thing for sure: I am just as strong as forty years ago."

An alcoholic patient had considerable difficulties with his family and his profession. When I asked him, "How are you?" I always received the same answer: "No change." This game of question and answer had become a ritual. I had the impression that it was fun for him to show that one couldn't achieve much with him. Whenever I brought up this subject in our therapy sessions, the patient avoided it. One day, after we had again conducted our ritual, I told him the story "I'm just as strong as forty years ago."

This story represented symbolicaliy the alcoholic's tendency to

136

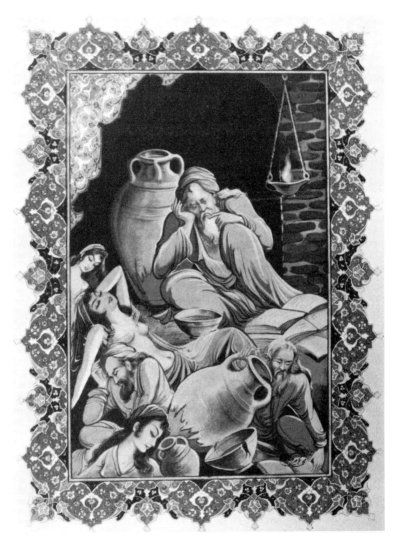

avoid his reality and sacrifice himself to unrealistic assertions. He was able to identify with the hero immediately. A seemingly immaterial, but nevertheless very symptomatic effect took place: The patient stopped using his stereotyped answer, "Things haven't changed with me." Instead, he tried to describe his actual state in a more differentiated way.

When King Amirnuhe Samani died, the scholars took the opportunity to conspire against Avicena, whom they considered a nuisance. As a result, Avicena had no choice but to leave the city of Gorgan and move to Rey, which belonged to the Dailamin dynasty. Rey was under the rule of King Madzdeldowleh. The ruler suffered terribly from severe melancholy and anorexia. Avicena was able to help him by using an unusual method. The ancient Persian poet Nizami describes the cure in this way:

The Cured Delusion

A ruler thought he was a cow and had completely forgotten that he was a human being. So he roared like an ox and begged, "Come; take me away, slaughter me, and make use of my flesh." Sending back all the food that was brought to him, he ate nothing. "Why don't you take me out to the green pastures so I can eat the way a cow should?" he asked. Since he no longer ate anything, he continually lost weight until he was nothing but a skeleton.

Since no methods or medications helped, Avicena was called in to give advice. He had it reported to the king that a butcher was coming to slaughter him, cut up his flesh, and give it to the people to eat. When the sick man heard this, he was happy beyond all measure and longingly waited for his death. On the appointed day, Avicena approached the king. He swung the butcher knife and screamed with a terrifying voice, "Where is the cow so I can finally slaughter it?" The king uttered a moo so the butcher would know where the sacrificial animal was. Then Avicena commanded loudly, "Bring the animal here; tie it down so I can chop off its head." But, before he swung with the knife he checked the loins and stomach of the animal for meat and fat, as butchers commonly do. But then he cried out with a loud voice, "No, no, this cow isn't mature enough to be slaughtered.

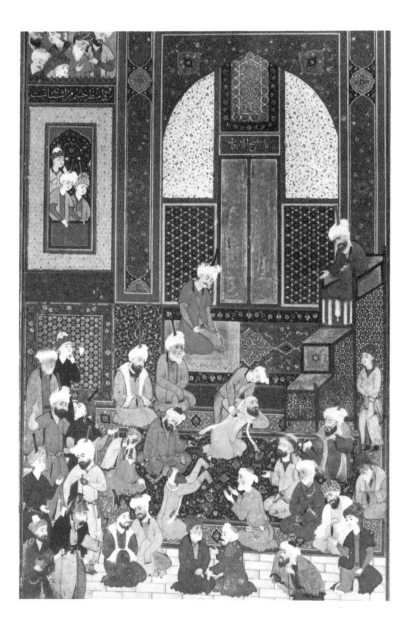

It's much too thin. Take it away and fatten it up. When it is at the right weight, I'll come again." The sick man ate every dish that was set before him, for he hoped to be slaughtered soon. He gained weight, his condition showed visible improvement, and he regained his health under Avicena's care.

I once had a fifty-one-year-old female patient whose illness had once been diagnosed as the defect of a paranoid-hallucinatory psychosis, and another time as chronic delusion. She reported, ". . . At first they blew and always blew it so that I always think about it, then they earlier, when the Rhine had dried up, they held Mao Tse-tung on my head and Professor Chap from Vietnam, and they always cried Lucifer. I checked that out, so that it must really be. Then they grew loud because of the Vietnam War where they double the roll, every day the bombs. That's how they always screamed. That was an eternity ago. You wouldn't believe what a terror that is. They got me onto the operating table—I don't know how often. Operations on my child, child torture, my father in the graveyard, my husband operated on; that's something, too. And that's why I want it to go to court. I've filed a complaint against them eight times. All they did was send me to a psychiatrist, that's all. Where there is all this evidence against them, a real pretext, and I sued them, at the work court, and then I found a lawyer, but I don't know, I hope that gets going now. I don't want to be persecuted the rest of my life by stupid, drunken, fucking Catholics. They're pious bigots, pious people in their modest clothes, kneeling beside me in church every Sunday. If I'd known that, I would have killed them. And the preacher always said to us at home just what they say here: The suffering is sent by God to make amends for our sins, and all the illnesses. Even a child has original sin and has to pay for it by being sick. There you stand, these idiots in the church. My mother sits there and prays. When I was there, I asked her why she was praying. Thanks for the food. You've already taken care of that, but she still prays silently. They caused her to have a heart attack, they beat on her heart so much. They did that to my child, too, even before he could walk and talk, and that for three generations. And now they're all about to lose. I hope the trial gets going now and that they hang them. And even if they say a hundred times that I'm nuts, the people in W——— wouldn't believe that at all, absolutely not. . . ."

Even if this text seems confused at first, very concrete experiences can be drawn and developed from it, assuming, of course, that one disregards the confused arrangement of the words and concentrates on the underlying rules for reproducing experiences. For this fifty-one-year-old patient, a strong need for justice forms the background for her statements. In one case, the justice refers to her profession, at another time to religion, then to sex, humanity, politics, doctors, her parents, the children, her husband, and so forth. "Justice" is her main theme, and around it are clustered a number of experienced situations of justice. It seems as if a "justice program" were running its course, at times not checked by reality.

If one examines the patient's past history and is guided by the actualizing capabilities, the partially dissociated utterances take on a plausible meaning. To put it briefly: The patient felt unjustly treated by all these institutions and people—and was certainly mistreated by them. Now she used her "delusion" to denounce these injustices. During the inventory of psychosocial impulses done with the aid of our differentiation analytical inventory (DAI), she replied completely logically and relevantly to the questions about the actual capabilities. Only when her repertoire was exhausted, did her "Justice program" begin to play again. The DAI made it possible for the patient to acquire a very differentiated self-image, one which would have been considered impossible, based on her deluded descriptions.

Although the patient's conviction about the world's injustice was almost unshakable, we were able to break down her delusion step by step. Of course, she would have hardly tolerated direct opposition. As the psychotherapist treating her, I would have immediately been seen as a member of that unjust world. So, the treatment took place via the analysis of the areas of conflict and the situations of justice linked with them. I tried to take part in the world of her experiences so I would understand them and could

141

then convey this understanding to the patient. Avicena had done something similar, and this method is clarified in modern psychotherapy, for example, by Benedetti (1976).

The willfulness of the illusory ideas, however, makes it hard for us to understand the hallucinatory patient and his utterances. As a result, the isolation of the patient and of his world increases. For the therapeutic process, it is all the more important that there be identification with the patient's experiences and thoughts, regardless of how strange they seem to us. Insofar as a general identification causes difficulties and is even something threatening for the therapist, a partial identification with the contents under consideration has proved to be useful.

The patient reacted very angrily and negatively when she just sensed an attempt to question her system of thought. But it was possible for her to laugh about her delusions and to talk about them in a distanced manner after I had told her a story about "Justice."

A Wise Judge

A woman who was very upset came to the ghazi, the circuit judge, and complained that a strange man had used force to try to kiss her. The woman cried out, "I demand justice from you. I won't have a moment's peace until you punish the wrongdoer. I demand it of you. It is my right." With these words, she stamped her foot vehemently and gave the judge an angry look. He was a wise man. He thought about it a long time and then pronounced the judgment. "You have been treated unjustly. You should therefore receive justice. The man kissed you forcefully and against your wishes. So that justice prevails, my judgment is, you should kiss him forcefully, too, and against his will." Turning to the bailiff, he ordered that the man be fetched so he could receive his punishment.

The patient had listened with wide open eyes and laughed out loud at the story's joke. It was all the more easy for her to get involved in the story, since the concept of justice in it was also linked to its sexual contents. At the following sessions, the patient again spoke about the story. Whenever the discussions about justice

142

reached a critical point for the patient, she built a bridge to the story, which, from all appearances, made it more bearable for her to examine critically her "illusion of justice."

Another Long Program

A merchant had a hundred and fifty camels to carry his things, and forty servants who did as he ordered. One evening, he invited a friend, (Saadi) to join him. The whole night, he couldn't get any rest and talked constantly about his problems, troubles, and the rat race of his profession. He told of his wealth in Turkestan, spoke of his estates in India, and displayed his jewels and the titles to his lands. "O Saadi," he sighed, "I have another trip coming up. After this trip, I want to settle back and have a hard-earned rest. That's what I want more than anything in the world. I want to take Persian sulphur to China, since I've heard that it is very valuable there. From there I want to transport Chinese vases to Rome. My ship will then carry Roman goods to India, and from there I will take Indian steel to Halab. From there, I will export mirrors and glass to Yemen and take velvet into Persia." With a sad expression on his face, he then proclaimed to Saadi, who had been listening in disbelief, "And, after that, my life will belong to peace, reflection, and meditation, the highest goal of my thoughts."

(After Saadi)

A forty-eight-year-old-man, the owner of a large factory with some hundred employees, had brought his two children to me for therapy. He said they had poor concentration, problems in school, and caused a lot of grief for their parents . Even if these complaints were justified, the man's statements gave me the impression that he was using the children as an excuse to allude to his own problems. He seemed frantic and anxious. This impression was confirmed the minute we stopped talking about the children and began to talk about him. It was as if a barrel had been opened up. With strong emotional involvement, interrupted by crying, he talked about himself, his problems, and the apparent hopelessness of his situation. He concluded by saying he wanted to be a patient, too.

143

Although he could point to economic success, he kept repeating, "I am a derelict. I have accomplished nothing."

These utterances, of course, could have just been the coquetry of a successful man who was boasting behind his modesty. Even if this element were present, the emotional crisis the patient described seemed serious enough. He had taken over the company from his father, who, as a self-made man, had built it up from nothing. His motto had been "Man must eat his bread from the sweat of his brow." Originally the patient had wanted a different career for himself. He had wanted to be an architect. But his father had canceled that idea. Again and again, the father had reminded his sons that he had done all this hard work for them and had built up the company just for them. This moral appeal to take over the father's inheritance was something the patient could not escape.

Then the father died suddenly, before the patient had really established himself in the firm. The patient was thus burdened with responsibility for the company and the need to be capable of doing it. As long as he shared the work with his brother, he was more or less on top of things. But then his brother died, too, in a car accident, and the patient was left with all responsibility for the business.

With his father's example in mind, the patient placed extraordinary demands on himself. To prove to himself that he was able to run the company as well as his father had done, he fired competent workers, took over their areas of responsibility, and demanded more and more of himself. This compulsion to achieve also entered his private life. Since he couldn't handle everything at work, he brought home reports, bills, and business documents so he could work on them there. Aside from this collision with the interests of his family, he became farther behind with his work and finally began to react in the opposite way. He suddenly refused to deal with all the professional demands, stopped going to his office, and stayed in bed. He brooded a lot, became overly sensitive, and had strong emotional outbursts at the slightest mention of his firm, his father, and his brother. Fighting back the tears, he would say, "I am at my wit's end. I don't know what I should do. I am completely wiped out."

It was strange that the patient had chosen this particular time to expand the company and erect new buildings valued at several million dollars. He explained this paradox by saying he would really prefer to retire from the business and enjoy some peace and quiet, but he owed it to his children, of course, to increase the family estate, which they would one day inherit. The obvious contradictions were, so it seems, not yet apparent to the patient. For this reason, I told him, almost in passing, the story, "Another Long Program," which Saadi told in his book *Golestan*. This story is acutally a caricature, but aptly depicts the hectic pace and the extreme activity, as well as the inconsistency that plagued the patient.

He recognized himself in the story immediately. It was the starting point for several conversations in which we dealt with ambition and achievement, the influence of the patient's image of his father, and the patient's excessive demands on himself. Step by step, we approached the problem of the patient's identification with his father and his desperate attempt to live up to his idealized view of the man. But there were strong objections to dealing with this theme, for the patient held rigid ideas about his father, and now sought to convince his sons of their responsibilities to the company, certainly as a testament to his own problems. At the same time, he repeatedly emphasized that he hated the company, that it hardly gave him the chance to be himself, and that he had neglected to live a life of his own, "just like the merchant in the story."

The goal of therapy was not to get the patient to avoid the demands of the business by delegating them, or to solve the organizational problems by simplifying the business and adopting more efficient procedures. Rather, the goal was to make the patient more aware of the conflict, his "struggle in the shadows," his strong emotional dependencies. For a long time, the central issue of the therapy was the patient's attempt to transfer his father image to me and to have me make all the decisions and bear the responsibilities. The patient became more and more aware of the discrepancy between the business, his motivation to achieve, and his own personal needs. In the final stages of the therapy, which involved the expansion of goals, attention to the contents, and an examination of previously neglected capabilities, I told him a story which described—indirectly, of course,—the patient's development during his treatment.

The Golden Tent Spikes

A dervish, whose joy was self-denial and whose hope was paradise, once met a prince, whose wealth exceeded everything the dervish had ever seen. The nobleman's tent, pitched outside the city for recreation, was made of precious fabrics, and even the spikes that held it up were solid gold. The dervish,who was used to preaching asceticism, attacked the prince with a flood of words about the futility of earthly wealth, the vanity of the golden tent spikes, and the fruitlessness of human endeavor. How eternal and majestic, on the other hand, were the holy places. Resignation, he said, was the greatest happiness. The prince listened seriously and with great thought. He took the dervish's hand and said, "For me your words are like the fire of the midday sun and the clarity of the evening breeze. Friend, come with me, accompany me on the way to the holy places." Without looking back, without taking money or a servant, the prince set out on the way.

Astonished,the dervish hurried along behind him. "Lord," he cried, "tell me, are you really serious about making a pilgrimage to the holy places? If you are, wait for me so I can go get my pilgrim's cloak."

Smiling kindly, the prince answered, "I left behind my wealth, my horses, my gold, my tent, my servants, and everything I owned. Do you have to go back just because of your cloak?" "Lord," replied the dervish with surprise, "please explain to me—how you could leave all your treasures behind and even go without your princely cloak?"

The prince spoke slowly but with a steady voice, "We sank the golden tent spikes into the earth, but not into our heart."

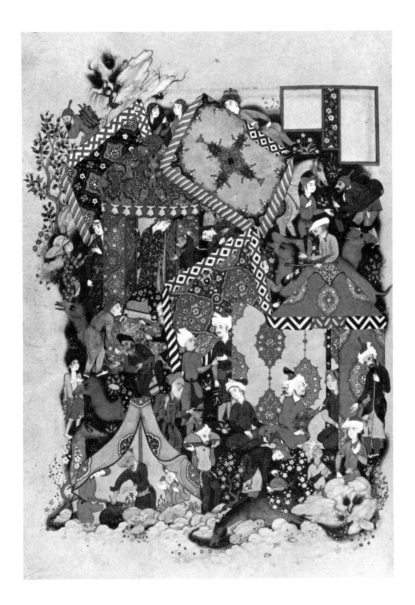

5.

A Collection of Stories to Think About

Here we present some stories without interpretations. The reader can interpret these stories for himself, try to find what they have to say, and share his interpretations with his spouse, his family, or other people. In so doing, he will discover two things: In many respects, all the interpretations will be similar. But, on the other hand, many ideas will be grasped differently, depending on the point of view the person takes. To the extent that the interpretations are also personal points of view, reflecting the reader's own situation, conversations about the stories and their interpretations can also be a method of self-discovery.

The Difficulty of Doing Things Right for Everyone

In the heat of the day, a father went through the dusty streets of Keshan with his son and a donkey. The father sat on the donkey, and the boy led it. "The poor kid," said a passer-by. "His short little legs try to keep up with the donkey. How can that man sit there so lazily on the donkey when he sees that the boy is running himself ragged." The father took this comment to heart, climbed down from the donkey at the next corner, and let the boy climb up. But it wasn't long before a passer-by again raised his voice and said, "What a disgrace! The little brat sits up there like a sultan, while his poor old father runs alongside." This remark hurt the boy very

148

much, and he asked his father to sit behind him on the donkey. "Have you ever seen anything like that," griped a veiled woman. "Such cruelty to animals. The poor donkey's back is sagging, and that old good-for-nothing and his son lounge around as if it were a divan—the poor creature!" The targets of this criticism looked at each other and, without saying a word, climbed down from the donkey. But they had barely gone a few steps when a stranger poked fun at them by saying, "Thank heavens I'm not that stupid. Why do you two walk your donkey when he doesn't do you any good, when he doesn't even carry one of you?" The father shoved a handful of straw into the donkey's mouth and laid his hand on his son's shoulder. "Regardless of what we do," he said, "there's someone who disagrees with it. I think we have to know for ourselves what we think is right."

The Sewer Cleaner's Attar of Roses

A sewer cleaner who had spent his whole life clearing out the city's sewage and transporting it to the surrounding fields came to the bazaar one day. In the course of time, he had gotten used to the horrible smell of the sewage. Without being disturbed, he could bravely walk through the town's sewage dumps, and, without wrinkling his nose, empty out the deepest sewage ditches. Now when the good man went through the alleys of the bazaar—they had never seen him there before—he came to a booth where a merchant sold attar of roses. The fragrance, which everyone else finds so wonderful, was so overpowering that the sewer cleaner fainted. All the attempts to arouse him proved fruitless. The people all stood around the unconscious man, not knowing what to do. A hakim, recognizing the man's profession by his clothing, grabbed a hunk of mud from the street and held it under the man's nose. Suddenly, as if touched by a magic wand, the sewer cleaner opened his eyes. The spectators stared, dumbfounded at this miracle. But the hakim said nonchalantly, "The man was not familiar with the fragrance of the attar of roses. His attar of roses is made of other material. How can he who has discovered nothing about being, know what being is?"

(After Saadi)

What a Person Has, He Has

A believer knelt in a mosque, deep in prayer. Someone near him was struck by his wonderful, artfully woven, pointed-toed shoes, called giwees. The man imagined how nice it would be to have shoes like that, too. The step from thought to deed is often smaller than one thinks. He approached the praying man from behind and whispered into his ear, "Don't you know that prayers spoken with shoes on do not reach God's ear?" The believer interrupted his prayer and whispered back just as softly, "Well, if my prayer is not heard, at least I will still have my shoes."

The Memory Prop

In the hotter regions of Iran, the drinking water is one of the valuable things in life. It is collected in special cisterns and often carried in large jugs across great distances. A father sent his son to fetch water. "My son," he said, "take this jug and get us some water, but take care not to drop the jug and spill the water." With these words, he extended his arm and gave his son a resounding slap to the side of the head. Eyes filled with tears, but still clutching the jug, the son went to the cistern. "Why did you hit our child," asked the mother angrily. "He didn't do anything." To this the father replied, "This slap will be a memory prop for him. I tell you, his whole life long he will never dare drop a jug with water in it. What good would it do if I slapped him after he had perhaps already shattered the jug?"

The Reward for Cleanliness

A man once had a wife who was known as a fanatical housekeeper. She had nothing better to do than chase every speck of dust in the house and polish every piece of furniture, even the earthen spittoon in the corner. But in the course of all her housework she completely neglected herself and ran around looking terribly unkempt. When her husband finally returned from a long trip one day, he felt the need to spit and thus clear his throat of all the dust he had breathed during the trip. Looking around, he tried to find the dirtiest corner in the house so that he could spit into it. But everything sparkled from cleanliness. So there was nothing he could do but spit in his wife's face.

About Eternal Life

During the time that the Prophet Mohammed was born, King Anoschirwan, whom the people also called "The Just," traveled through his kingdom. On a sunny slope, he saw a venerable old man bent over, hard at work. Followed by his courtiers, the king came nearer and saw that the old man was planting year-old seedlings. "What are you doing there?" the king inquired.

"I'm planting nut trees," replied the man.

The king asked in amazement, "You are already quite old. Why are you planting seedlings when you won't see their foliage, won't rest in their shade, and won't eat their fruit?" The old man looked up and said, "Those who came before us planted, and we were able to harvest. Now we plant so that they who come after us can harvest."

The Divided Duties

"I can't take it any longer. The tasks are like mountains that I can no longer move. Early in the morning I have to wake you up, straighten up the house, clean the carpets, look after the children, shop at the bazaar, cook your favorite rice dish for supper, and then still pamper you at night." This is what a woman said to her husband.

Chewing on a chicken leg, he simply said, "What's so bad about that? All women do what you do. You've got it good. While I bear all sorts of responsibilities, you just sit around at home."

"Oh," complained the wife, "if only you could help me a bit." Overcome by generosity, the man finally agreed to the following suggestion: While his wife would take responsibility for everything that happened in the house, he would take over all the tasks outside the house. This division of tasks enabled the couple to live together contentedly for a long time.

One day the husband went shopping with friends and then sat in a coffee shop, contentedly smoking a waterpipe. Suddenly, a neighbor rushed in and cried out excitedly, "Hurry, your house is burning."

The man continued smoking on the waterpipe and said with marvelous indifference, "Be so good as to tell my wife, since she has final say for everything that happens in the house. I'm responsible only for outside duty."

151

The Wisdom of the Master

A pupil once came to a well-known wrestling champion to be instructed in the art of wrestling. For years he practiced with the greatest zeal and the most admirable talent. "Master," he asked one day, "is there anything left that you can still teach me?"

"You have learned everything I could teach," the master said. These words made the young wrestler feel so proud that he proclaimed throughout the land that he was now the best one and could even defeat the famous champion. Thousands of people came to watch the match between the two. After a long, evenly matched contest, the master suddenly shouldered his pupil with a surprising hold and defeated him.

"Strange," said the pupil, choking, "I learned everything from you. How did you happen to overwhelm me with a hold that I did not know?"

"Young friend," said the champion, "it's right. I taught you everything I could. But I kept this single hold for myself until today."

(After Saadi)

Late Revenge

A man was punished by his fellow-villagers by being thrown into a dry cistern. The townspeople who had been treated unjustly by him now took justice into their own hands. They stood at the rim of the ditch and unleashed a shower of spit upon the man. Others threw mud from the street. Suddenly the man was hit by a stone. In amazement, he looked up and asked the stone-thrower, "I know all the other people. Who are you, that you think you can throw stones at me?"

The man up on the edge of the ditch replied, "I'm the man you treated badly twenty years ago."

The sinner then asked, "Where were you all this time?" "The whole time," the man answered, "I carried the stone in my heart. Now that I found you in such a wretched condition, I took the stone in my hand."

The Dark Side of the Sun

Every day, a scholar came to the Prophet Mohammed. One day the prophet took him aside and said, "So that our love will grow, I don't want you to come here every day." Then Mohammed told of this incident: A scholar was once asked, "The sun is so majestic and wonderful, and yet we never hear of someone loving it in particular." The scholar answered, "The sun shines on us every day. And only in winter do we cherish it, because then it hides behind the clouds."

A Good Business

"Get up, Badmazhab, you godless creature," scolded a Bedouin as he beat with his club on a camel which was kneeling lazily and defiantly in the sand. "If you again ignore my words, I will sell you at the bazaar for a tuman {fifty cents}, you worthless creature, I swear it by Allah." But not even a whole day passed and the Bedouin again had to beat the lazy animal. What the man had sworn had now occurred. He would have to keep his promise. Quarreling with himself, with the camel, and with God, he brought the animal to the bazaar to sell it. He regretted his hasty promise. One tuman for a camel was much too little. He should have sworn to sell it for a hundred. But suddenly he had an idea of how he could save himself. He ran home and got his old, half-blind cat. He tied it to the camel and cried out at the bazaar, "A marvelous camel for a tuman. Come buy it, folks. You'll never again see an offer like this. A camel for a tuman." But when someone showed interest in it, the Bedouin said cunningly, "The camel costs only a tuman. But I will only sell it along with the cat, and it costs ninty-nine tuman." Until evening came, the Bedouin extolled the camel with its expensive supplement. A large crowd of people gathered around and laughed about the Bedouin's cunning salesmanship, but no one wanted to buy the camel. That evening, the Bedouin went home satisfied, leading the camel and the cat on a line. He said to himself, "I swore to sell the camel for a tuman. I did everything to keep my promise, but the people just didn't like the idea. Let them be punished for the fact that my oath was not carried out, the godless old skinflints!"

Theory and Practice of Knowing People

An intelligent young man, thirsty for knowledge and wisdom, had studied physiognomy, the science of deducing temperament from outward appearance. His studies, which lasted six years, took place in Egypt and cost him many sacrifices far from his homeland. But finally he completed his exams with excellent results. Filled with pride and joy, he rode back to his home. Everyone he met on the way he looked at with the eyes of his science, and, in order to extend his knowledge, he read the facial expressions of all the people he encountered.

One day he met a man whose face was stamped by six qualities: envy, jealousy, greed, covetousness, stinginess, and inconsideration. "My God, what a monstrous expression! I've never seen or heard of anything like that before. I could test my theory here."

While he was thinking this, the stranger approached with a friendly, kind, and modest demeanor, saying "Oh sheik. It is already very late and the next village is far away. My cottage is small and dark, but I will carry you in my arms. What an honor it would be for me if I could consider you my guest for the night. And how happy I would be in your presence!"

Amazed by this, the traveler thought to himself, "How astonishing! What a difference between this stranger's speech and his horrible facial expression." This realization frightened him very much. He began to doubt the things he had learned in the past six years. In order to gain some certainty, he accepted the stranger's invitation. The man pampered the scholar with tea, coffee, fruit juices, pastries, and a waterpipe. He overwhelmed his guest with kindness, with attention, goodness, and politeness. For three days and three nights, the host succeeded in keeping our traveler there. Eventually the scholar was able to resist his host's politeness. He firmly decided to continue his journey. When the time had come for him to leave, his host handed him an envelope and said, "O lord. Here is your bill."

"What bill?" the scholar asked, surprised.

As fast as a person can draw a sword form its sheath, the host suddenly showed his true face. He wrinkled his brow sternly and screamed with an angry voice, "What impudence! What were you thinking when you ate everything here? Did you think it was all free?" Upon hearing these words, the scholar suddenly came to his senses. Without saying a word, he opened the letter. There he saw that everything he had eaten and not eaten had been billed to him a hundred times over. He did not even have half the money that was demanded of him. Forced by necessity, he climbed down from his horse and gave it to his host. Then he took off his traveling clothes and set off on foot. As if in ecstasy, he bowed his torso with every step of the way. From far off, one could hear him saying, "Thank God, thank God my six years of study were not in vain!"

(After 'Abdu'l-Bahá)

The Value of a Pearl

In a garden a rooster saw an iridescent pearl hidden on the ground. He greedily pounced on it, dug it out, and tried to force it down his gullet. When he noticed that the shiny object was not the queen of the grains of rice, he spit the pearl out. He had certainly checked the pearl, but what kind of test was it! The pearl called to the rooster and said, "I am a lustrous, precious pearl. By chance I fell from a wonderful necklace and landed in this garden. There aren't pearls like me everywhere. Not every ocean has marvelous pearls like me. Only chance threw me at your feet. One doesn't find me like sand at the sea. If you would look at me with the eyes of reason, you would see thousands of wonders and beauties." But the rooster crowed with a proud voice, "I'd give you away if someone would just trade me a grain of rice."

(After P. Etessami, Persian Poet)

The Polite Mullah

Once again an esteemed sheik gave a big party. All the dignitaries of the town were invited, but not the mullah. Nevertheless, he was seen among the guests, feeling as at home as a fish in water. Somewhat shocked, a friend took him aside and said, "What are you doing here? You aren't invited!" Filled with lenience, the mullah answered, "If the host doesn't know his duty and doesn't invite me, why should I neglect my duty to be a polite guest?"

155

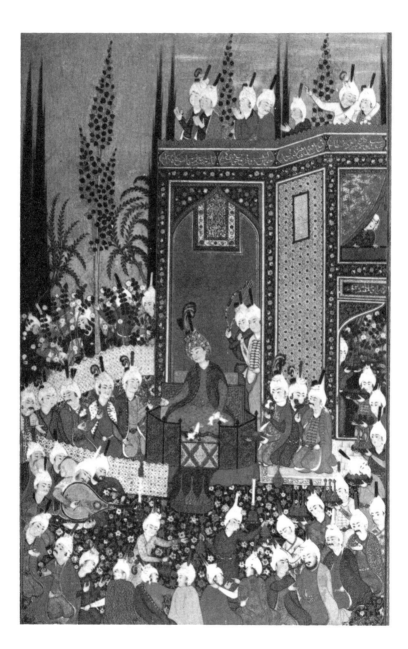

Biographical Sketches

Abdu'l-Bahá (1844–1921): Bahá'u'lláh's oldest son, designated by him as official spokesman for his teachings. Along with his father, he was exiled and imprisoned until 1908. During a three-year trip to Egypt, Europe, and North America, he spread the Baha'i religion and established contact with the important figures of his time.

Ali (600–661): Through marriage to Fatima he was Mohammed's son-in-law. His murder led to the break between Sunnites and Shiites, of whom he is considered to be the first Imam (follower of Mohammed). The Moslems of Iran are mostly Shiites.

Anowschirwan (ca. 530): He is regarded as the greatest king of the Sassanites and was known most of all for his justice. During his reign, the collection of stories *Kalilee we-Damaneh* was brought to Persia from India and was translated into the Pahlwi language.

Avicena (980–1037): A member of the nobility, he was a physician, philosopher, and diplomat. He wrote numerous philosophical and medical works. His *Canon of Medical Science,* in particular, influenced the development of European medicine.

Báb (1819–1850): Born in Shiraz. By appealing to the Holy Scriptures of earlier revelations, he lay claim to being the herald and forerunner of a new prophet. He is the precursor of the Bahá'i religion. Because of his religious claims, he was taken prisoner and executed in Tabriz. This marked the beginning of a massacre in which some twenty thousand Bábi (followers of Báb) were murdered.

Bahá'u'lláh (1817–1892): Founder of the Bahá'i religion of which Báb was the forerunner. He was eventually banished to the prison city of Akka. His banishment lasted twenty-four years. During this time, he wrote down his message. In more than one hundred documents, he explained the foundations of his faith.

Behaedine Ameli (ca. 1575): Known as Sheik Behai; he was a philosopher, physicist, and poet. Along with other books, one of the best-loved collections of maxims is his *Mouse and Cat,* in which he presents social criticism through the medium of fables.

Christ (beginning of the Christian record of time): Founder of Christianity. For thirty years, he lived in Nazareth, then traveled through the land as a wandering preacher and worker of miracles. Because of alleged blasphemy and supposed political danger, he was crucified. The New Testament of the Bible contains his works and his message.

Ettasami, Parwin (1906–1941): Daughter of the Persian writer Jussuf Etassami. Through poems in which she expressed views on various social issues, she struggled for recognition and equal rights for women. It was her goal to increase human ability to make decisions.

Hafis (1320?–1389?): After Saadi he is considered the most famous Persian poet. He spent his entire life in Shiraz. His most famous work is *Hafis' Divan,* which influenced Goethe's *Westöstliches Diwan.* During the period when the Mongolians invaded Persia, his stories became the chief vehicles of Persian culture.

Mohammed (570–632): The founder of Islam, he experienced his calling in 610 At the center of his revelations is the uniqueness of the God of Creation. Persecuted in Mecca, he migrated to Medina (Hedshra). His teachings are set forth in the Koran.

Mowlana (1248–1317): One of the chief mystics and poets of the Persian language. Because his complete name was Mowlana Djalaldine Rumi, many of his stories are listed under the name Rumi. His book *Massnawi* contains forty-seven thousand poems. It is dedicated to the Sufi Schams, from whom we have taken "The Miracle of the Ruby."

Razi (850–923): He was one of the great Persian physicians, uniting the knowledge of Greek and Arabic medicine. Instead of limiting himself to theory, he recorded his own observations about such things as smallpox, measles, and gallstones.

Saadi (1211–1300): His most important book is *Golestan* (Flower garden), which presents the poems he wrote during the forty years of pilgrimage which took him to Iran, India, Arabia, and North Africa. His poems and proverbs have become a part of Iranian folklore and are treasured as practical aids in daily life. He was known as the teacher of teachers.

Solomon (972–929 BC.): Son of David, the third king of Israel, who brought its power to its greatest height, was known most of all for building the temple in Jerusalem. The *Book of Proverbs,* The *Song of Solomon,* and the *Book of Wisdom* are attributed to Solomon.

Bibliography

English

Baha'u'llah: *Gleanings from the Writings of Baha'u'llah*
—— *Seven Valleys. 1975.*
Fromm, E.: *Escape from Freedom. New York. 1941.*
—— "The Oedipus Complex and the Oedipus Myth," 1949. In: Anshen, R. N.:
   The Family: Its functions and Destiny. New York, 1949.
Gifford, E. W.: *Mohave and Yuma Indians,* cited in R. Wood, *World of Dreams; An
   Anthology.* New York 1947.
James, W.: *The Dilemma of Determinism,* first published in 1884.
Jung, C. G.: *Memories, Dreams, Reflections.* New York, 1963.
Peseschkian, N.: *In Search of Meaning. A Psychotherapy of Small Steps.* Berlin
   Heidelberg New York Tokyo, 1985.
—— *Psychotherapy of Everyday Life. Training in Partnership and Self-Help.* Berlin
   Heidelberg New York Tokyo, 1986.
—— *Positive Family Therapy. The Family as Therapist.* Berlin Heidelberg
   New York Tokyo, 1986.
—— *Positive Psychotherapy.* Berlin Heidelberg New York Tokyo (in preparation).
—— *Positive Psychotherapy in Psychosomatics.* Berlin Heidelberg New York
   (in preparation).

German

Abdu'l Baha: *Beantwortete Fragen.* Frankfurt, 1962.
Ackerknecht, E. H.: *Geschichte der Medizin.* Stuttgart 1955.
Andrae, T.: *Islamische Mystiker.* Stuttgart, 1960.
Battegay, R.: *Narzismus und Objektbeziehungen: über das Selbst zum Objekt.* Bern,
   1977.
Benedetti, G.: *Der Geisteskranke als Mitmensch.* Göttingen, 1976.

161

Daschti, A.: *Über Hafis* (persisch). Teheran, 1958.

Etessami, P.: *Diwan* (Gesamtwerk, persisch). Teheran, 1954.

Fetscher, I.: *Wer hat Dornröschen wachgeküßt? Das Märchenverwirrbuch.* Frankfurt 1972.

Freud, S.: *Der Witz und seine Beziehung zum Unbewußten,* Gesammelte Werke, Bd. VI. Frankfurt, 1973.

Fromm E.: *Märchen, Mythen and Träume.* Zürich, 1957.

Ghowharin, S.: *Biographie über Avicena* (persisch). Teheran, 1953.

Goeppert, S.: "Vom Nutzen der Psychoanalyse für die Literaturkritik." *Confinia psychiat,* 20:95–107, 1977.

Meves, Chr.: *Erziehen und erzählen: über Kinder und Märchen.* Berlin, 1971.

Meyer-Steineg, Th., Sudhoff, K.: *Geschichte der Medizin im Überblick.* Jena, 1921.

Mowlana, Massnavi: *Gesamtwerk.* Teheran, 1960.

Peseschkian, N.: *Positive Psychotherapie: Theorie und Praxis einer neuen Methode.* Frankfurt, 1977.

———— *Schatten auf der Sonnenuhr, Erziehung, Selbsthilfe Psychotherapie.* Wiesbaden, 1974.

———— *Psychotherapie des Alltagslebens: Training zu Partnerschaftserziehung und Selbsthilfe.* Frankfurt, 1977.

———— *Auf der Suche nach Sinn. Frankfurt, 1983.*

———— *Positive Familientherapie. Eine Behandlungsmethode der Zukunft.* Frankfurt, 1980.

Saadi: *Gholestan* (persisch). Teheran, 1953.

Sager, C.J., Kaplan, H.S. (Hrsg.): *Handbuch der Ehe-, Familien- und Gruppentherapie,* 3. Bd. München, 1973.

Schnütgen, W.: *"Die Kalifen und ihre Ärzte". Naturheilkunde,* Heft 4, April, 1978.

Towhidipour, M. (Hrsg.): *Maus und Katze von Scheich Behai* (persisch). Teheran, 1958.

Watzlawick, P., Beavin, J.H., Jackson, D.D.: *Menschliche Kommunikation: Formen, Störungen, Paradoxien.* Bern, 1969.

———— Weakland, J.H., Fisch, R.: Lösungen: *zur Theorie und Praxis menschlichen Wandels,* Bern. 1974.

Wolpe, J.: *Praxis der Verhaltenstherapie.* Bern, 1972.

Index

166

Six important books by N. Peseschkian

N. Peseschkian

Oriental Stories as Tools in Psychotherapy

The Merchant and the Parrot
1st edition. 1982. Corrected 2nd printing 1986. 15 figures. 192 pages
ISBN 3-540-15765-4

Oriental Stories as Tools in Psychotherapy represents a new approach that taps fantasy and intuition and reactivates the individual's potential for conflict-solving.

N. Peseschkian

Positive Family Therapy

The Family as Therapist
Translated from the German by M. Rohlfing
1986. Approx. 340 pages. ISBN 3-540-15768-9

Positive Family Therapy focuses on the given capacity of the family as a whole to deal with conflicts within the family and the afflications of its members through group discussion.

N. Peseschkian

Psychotherapy of Everyday Life

Training in Partnership and Selfhelp
With 250 Case Histories
1986. Approx. 10 figures. Approx. 240 pages. ISBN 3-540-15767-0

Psychotherapy of Everyday Life illustrates day-to-day conflicts that occur in partnerships, how they can arise from misunderstandings and how the layman can deal with them.

N. Peseschkian

In Search of Meaning

A Psychotherapy of Small Steps
1985. 25 figures. 216 pages. ISBN 3-540-15766-2

In Search of Meaning shows that individuals suffering from a loss of meaning cannot find what they are looking for in a global concept, but rather must first take small steps to find the meaning behind single actions.

N. Peseschkian

Positive Psychotherapy

1986. ISBN 3-540-15794-8

N. Peseschkian

Positive Psychotherapy in Psychosomatics

1986. ISBN 3-540-15769-7

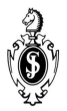

Springer-Verlag
Berlin
Heidelberg
New York
Tokyo